DATE DUE

3/18/96			
MAR 1 0 1999			
APR 0 1 1999			
MAY 1 4 1999			
MY 1 0 '99			
MAY 1 4 1999			
DEC 1 7 1999			
12-7-00			
DE 12 '00			
GAYLORD			PRINTED IN U.S.A.

Teenage
and
Pregnant

WHAT YOU CAN DO

Herma Silverstein

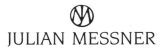

JULIAN MESSNER

Published by Julian Messner, a division of
Silver Burdett Press, Inc., Simon & Schuster, Inc.,
Prentice Hall Bldg., Englewood Cliffs, NJ 07632.

JULIAN MESSNER and colophon are trademarks of
Simon & Schuster, Inc. Design by Iris Weinstein
Manufactured in the United States of America.
(Lib. ed.) 10 9 8 7 6 5 4 3 2
(Paper ed.) 10 9 8 7 6 5 4

Library of Congress Cataloging-in-Publication Data

Silverstein, Herma.
    Teenage and pregnant : what you can do / Herma Silverstein.
        p. cm.
    Bibliography: p.
    Includes index.
    Summary: A handbook presenting the options available to a
teenage girl who finds herself pregnant. Includes information on
legal rights, the birth process, parenthood, adoption procedures,
programs for young mothers, and school and employment training.
    1. Teenage pregnancy—United States—Juvenile literature.
2. Pregnant schoolgirls—United States—Juvenile literature.
[1. Pregnancy.]   I. Title.
HQ759.4.S54   1988
306.7'088055—dc19   88–23087
                                                                   CIP
                                                                    AC
ISBN 0–671–65221–4 (lib. bdg.)
ISBN 0–671–65222–2 (pbk.)

To every teenager who has ever been pregnant and faced with monumentally difficult decisions, my wishes for your happiness and peace of mind—HS

Contents

Acknowledgments

I WISH TO THANK the following people and organizations for their dedication to the well-being of children and young adults and for their invaluable and enthusiastic assistance in providing me with material for this book:

Teresa Hauser, Ellen Reardon, Ruby Piester, Linda Pelts, William Hummer, M.D., and Angela Diaz, M.D., of the Mount Sinai Adolescent Health Center, New York City.

The U.S. Department of Health and Human Services; the March of Dimes Birth Defects Foundation; the Child Welfare League of America; the Children's Defense Fund; the Edna Gladney Maternity Home, Fort Worth, Texas; Saint Anne's Maternity Home, Los Angeles, California; Saint Peter Home for Children, Memphis, Tennessee; the Alan Guttmacher Institute; Planned Parenthood Federation of America; the National Committee for Adoption; Adoption Services of Western Association of Concerned Adoptive Parents; Services for Unmarried Parents and Specialized Adoptions; the

Acknowledgments

Charles Stewart Mott Foundation; the National Family Planning and Reproductive Health Association; Concerned United Birthparents; the University of Utah Medical Center, Blackstone; and Comtois & Assoc.

ONE

I Thought It Couldn't Happen to Me

CATHY SAT on her bed staring at the phone on her night table. Two months had gone by since her last period. And for the past few weeks she'd awakened every morning so sick to her stomach she'd barely made it into the bathroom before throwing up. What if she was really pregnant?

But she couldn't be. They'd only had sex that one time. Cathy reached for the phone, then stopped. What would Tim say when she told him? He said he loved her and wanted to marry her—when they were older. Not now, when they still had two years of high school left. Cathy sank down on her bed. What if Tim got mad at her for being pregnant— if she really was pregnant? What if he broke up with her? She'd be all alone, with a baby to take care of.

Cathy's stomach tightened as she thought about telling her parents. They'd probably yell at her. Tell her she was a terrible daughter. Maybe even kick her out of the house. Her father hadn't been well lately. What if he had a heart attack when she told him? Maybe she could get an abortion. But how? Where? And with what money?

She took a deep breath and tried to relax. Hey, what was she getting so upset about? She probably wasn't pregnant anyway. Her period was a month overdue, but that didn't mean she was pregnant. She was probably just irregular, like her sister. Yes, that must be it. Cathy sighed, relieved that she'd found the solution. Now she could forget all about it.

Maybe you or someone you know is having the same worry as Cathy. Most teenagers, when they suspect they are pregnant, try to deny it by making up other reasons for the early symptoms of pregnancy. These symptoms include missing a period, nausea and vomiting (more commonly called morning sickness), swollen or tender breasts, and a general feeling of being tired and sleepy all the time. Teenagers may tell themselves that morning sickness is a case of the flu and that they've missed a period just because their periods are irregular.

Denial stems from fear, either of the unknown or of something specific, such as "What will my parents say?". Denying something you know is true takes a lot of energy. The result is a feeling of being stressed out and depressed, which can lead to mental paralysis, an inability to take positive action to deal with an unpleasant situation. Thus, a girl might let months go by without having a pregnancy test or telling anyone of her suspicions. By then, the only option left could be to have the baby.

Ellen, fifteen, describes her reaction to being pregnant: "I was always a little overweight, and I'd go on these starvation diets and lose weight, then gain it back again. So I kept telling myself, 'I'm just gaining weight,' because I didn't want to believe I was pregnant. Then I felt the baby move inside me, and I knew."

"I was so scared about telling my parents," another girl says. "I thought they'd kill me. Whenever I was in the room with them, I'd sort of slouch over and not look at them. I just knew they'd be able to tell I was pregnant by looking at me."

Carol, fourteen, says, "I was going to have an abortion. My boyfriend took me to the clinic, but I couldn't go through with it. I kept putting it off, and when I finally went to see a doctor, he told me it was too late to have an abortion. So I just put it far back in my mind and tried to forget about it."

And Tracy, seventeen, talks about the loneliness and despair that girls often feel when they keep their pregnancies secret: "I felt like I was at the bottom of a swimming pool with weights on my feet. I was drowning, and there was no one to call for help. Being pregnant is the hardest thing I've ever done. When you have a baby, you have to grow up fast."

For most girls, finding out they are pregnant comes as a shock, even if they have suspected it for some time. "It can't happen to me" or "There must be a mistake" are some common reactions to the news.

Michelle was eighteen and about to graduate from high school when she became pregnant. "When the doctor told me my pregnancy test came out positive, I said, 'What do you mean it came out positive?'. I walked out of his office in kind of a daze. It didn't really hit me until I was outside,

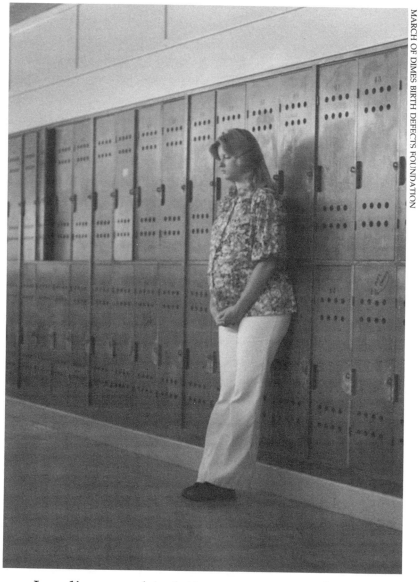

Loneliness and isolation are common feelings among pregnant teenagers.

and then I started crying and saying, 'Oh, my gosh. This can't happen to me.' I was walking down the street crying, and people were staring at me. I had my car, but I wasn't in any condition to drive."

When girls are as frightened as Michelle, they often do everything they can think of to hide their pregnancy. They almost seem to believe that if they don't think about being pregnant, the problem will go away. Some girls are able to postpone telling anyone for months.

"My folks didn't know I was pregnant until about the sixth month," says seventeen-year-old Teresa. "I was afraid of how mad they'd be when they found out, and I didn't want anyone telling me to get an abortion. So I just wore big shirts over my jeans. Then one day I was taking a bath, and my mom came into the room. When she saw how big my stomach was, there was no way I could hide it from her anymore."

Gwen, age fourteen, says, "I waited four months to get a pregnancy test. I just kept avoiding it. I stopped looking at myself in the mirror. And I still had my periods, only a little lighter. So I kept telling myself I was just gaining weight. But my mom sort of knew anyway, because of all the questions I was asking her, like 'What are varicose veins?' She knew I'd missed two periods, but I'd just say, 'No, no, I'm not pregnant.' I couldn't go to sleep at night, I was so nervous. I read books to get my mind off it. I read so many books while I was pregnant. I had all the symptoms, but I didn't want to acknowledge it. When I finally admitted it to my mom, she cried for a long time. But she was great. She stuck by me through the whole thing."

Amazing as it sounds, more than one girl has succeeded

in hiding her pregnancy until she actually went into labor. Christine is one such girl.

"I'm skinny anyway, so I didn't show that much. I guess my folks thought I'd just gained a little weight or something. The way they found out was one night I got these cramps, and at first I thought it was just a bad stomach ache. But then the pain got worse and worse. I started screaming. My folks thought it was my appendix, and they took me to the emergency room of the hospital. This doctor was examining me when all this water gushed out of me. Like I'd wet my pants, only there was tons of water. The doctor said, 'I don't believe this. Your water broke. You're having a baby.' Stevie was born about an hour later. I was pregnant all those nine months, but I just kept telling myself, "I'm not. I'm not.' "

Another girl says, "I completely denied I was pregnant even after I went into labor. I've always been heavy, and it was winter, so I just wore big sweaters all the time. Then I started having contractions. When they'd go away, I'd tell myself, 'Oh, good. I don't have to tell anyone yet.'

"Then the contractions got closer together, and they hurt a lot. My parents took me to the hospital because they didn't know what was wrong with me. The doctor heard the baby's heartbeat and told them. My mother almost went crazy. The nurses ran down the hall with me on this gurney, just like you see on television, banging through the double doors into the delivery room, and Sara was born a half-hour later. The next day a social worker came to talk to me, and I decided to put her up for adoption. It really went fast for me. I didn't have time to think about anything. It didn't hit me that I'd really had a baby until later."

Most girls, however, do tell someone before the baby arrives. When that person is a parent, reactions range from fear to shock, anger, embarrassment, and even happiness. Dolores, seventeen, was living with her sister when she became pregnant. "I didn't tell my parents at first," she says. "I just stopped calling them for two or three months. They figured something was wrong, and then when I did call, they were going, 'What's wrong? You didn't call for a long time.' I finally just told them. My dad blew up, yelling, 'How could you do this to me? We raised you to be a nice girl.' He was embarrassed to be seen with me. My mom was happy, I guess. At least she wasn't embarrassed like my dad."

When Jackie got pregnant, she was fifteen and studying to become a professional ballerina. "My parents were crushed. They said I'd really let them down, after they'd spent all that money on my ballet lessons. I felt so guilty. Now I'll probably never be a dancer, because I'll be too busy taking care of my baby."

Nancy, sixteen, was living with her boyfriend. "I was expecting to get pregnant, but when it happened and I told him, he split. I was scared, because I didn't know what to do. I couldn't afford to cover the rent by myself, so I moved back home. On Mother's Day I went into the kitchen to wish my mom a happy Mother's Day, and all of a sudden I blurted out that I was pregnant. She didn't yell and scream. She told me it was important to get good prenatal care. My dad stayed with me the whole time I was in the hospital. My parents were really supportive, and I'm living with them until I can take care of the baby myself."

For some girls who have steady boyfriends, there is a

feeling of joy in the idea of having a baby together. Their joy either remains or disappears, depending on their boy-friends' reaction to the pregnancy.

Trudy, eighteen, thought she had a great relationship with her boyfriend until she got pregnant. "Nick and I had talked about going to college, then finding good jobs and getting married. We were going to save up so we could have a house and money in the bank. But we never got that far, because I got pregnant, and he wanted nothing to do with me."

"Ron and I had always talked about having kids," another girl says. "So I couldn't wait to tell him I was pregnant. That was the last time I felt happy in nine months. I couldn't believe the way he acted. The first thing he said was, 'Are you sure it's mine?' That about killed me. Then he told me I'd have to get an abortion, that having a baby now would ruin his life. After that, he walked the other way whenever he saw me at school, and every time I call him now, his mom says he can't come to the phone."

Andrea's boyfriend had a slightly different reaction. "Carl didn't tell his parents until after I had the baby. His dad said, 'Deny everything. Don't put your name on any-thing.' So Carl said the baby wasn't his when it was time to sign the adoption papers, because if I changed my mind about the adoption, and his name was on papers saying he was the father, he might have to provide support for the baby. I envy the girls whose boyfriends stay with them. Before I got pregnant, Carl and I did everything together. Not anymore."

Rita, seventeen, had a happier outcome with her boy-friend. "Danny was so excited he couldn't stop grinning and hugging me. We went together to tell our folks. My mom kept crying, 'My baby's having a baby!' Both our parents wished we'd waited until we were older, but after they calmed down, they said they'd help us out financially if we stayed in school."

Girls like Andrea, Nancy, Ellen, and Cathy are part of a growing number of pregnant teenagers in the United States. Each day, an average of more than three thousand teenagers become pregnant, adding up to a total of 1.1 million a year. Almost eight out of ten of these girls are not married, and only one of those eight ends up marrying the father of the baby. Those who do marry are more likely to separate or divorce than couples who marry in their twenties.

These figures mean that one out of eleven girls age eleven to nineteen will become pregnant at least once before age twenty. If these figures continue to increase, according to the Alan Guttmacher Institute, soon four in ten girls will get pregnant while still in their teens. In fact, the teenage birthrate in the United States is higher than that of almost any other developed country.

Teenagers account for over one-fourth of the abortions performed in the United States each year, as about 40 percent of those 1.1 million pregnant girls get abortions. Of those who do not get abortions, only about 4 percent place their babies for adoption, while the remaining 96 percent keep their babies. Today there are approximately 1.3 million children living with 1.1 million teenage mothers, more than half of whom are single. These teenage mothers living alone, with little education or job skills, are five times as likely as women over twenty to be unemployed or to live below the poverty level. About one-fourth of teenage mothers receive welfare or Aid to Families with Dependent Children (AFDC).

The prospects for these girls to live above the poverty level are slim, as only 50 percent of those who give birth before age eighteen complete high school. Of girls who become mothers before age twenty, less than 2 percent complete college, and this makes it harder for them to get well-paid employment.

Although these figures sound bleak, there are ways to keep yourself from becoming another teenage pregnancy statistic. The most important way is to stay in school. *It is illegal for a school to expel a girl for being pregnant.* You are entitled to attend classes until you have your baby. In addition, many cities have special programs for pregnant or parenting teenagers. These programs often include prenatal and childbirth classes and day care facilities that take care of your child while you are in class. Check with your school counselor or look in the Yellow Pages under "Pregnancy" for the names of programs for pregnant teenagers in your area.

Why are there so many pregnant teenagers in the United States? Some girls take a chance on getting pregnant out of fear. A common fear is that they will "lose" the boy if they say no to sex. The fact is, however, that nine out of ten boys abandon a girl who gets pregnant. Other girls are afraid to use birth control for fear that if their friends find out they are sleeping with a boy, their reputations will be ruined. A girl may feel embarrassed about asking her boyfriend to use a condom, or she may be afraid that if she talks to her boyfriend about using contraception, he will think she routinely has sex with any boy she goes out with.

In addition to feeling afraid in these ways, many teenagers believe the myths they hear about how a girl gets pregnant. For instance, some teenagers believe that you cannot get pregnant the first time you have sex, or if you have sex only once. The fact is, however, that more than one-fifth of first pregnancies among teenagers occur in the first month after having sexual intercourse for the first time.

Other teenagers believe that if the girl takes a birth control pill just before having sex, she won't get pregnant. This is not true. Nor is it true that a girl cannot get pregnant if she has sex while standing up, or if she does not have an orgasm, or if she douches immediately afterward, or if the boy does not climax, or if he "pulls out" before climaxing.

Many girls mistakenly believe that if they have had sex several times without getting pregnant, this means they cannot get pregnant. The truth is that two-thirds of girls who have unprotected sex will get pregnant within two years.

Still other myths claim a girl cannot get pregnant if she is under twelve years old, has not yet had her first period, or is in the middle of her period, or if she urinates immediately afterward, or does some form of strenuous exercise after sex.

None of these myths are true. You can understand why they are untrue if you think about how a girl really does get pregnant.

Except when a girl is pregnant, her ovaries usually produce one egg a month, from puberty through menopause (around age forty-five to fifty-five). An egg is expelled from one ovary and then travels down the fallopian tube toward the uterus, which has been lining itself with blood and tissue in preparation for the possible fertilization of the egg. This journey takes about three days.

Fertilization occurs if the egg combines with a man's sperm. Then the fertilized egg divides until it is a tiny ball of cells, and plants itself into the uterus lining. The egg is now called an embryo until it is eight weeks old, at which point it is called a fetus. In the uterus, it grows and develops into a baby over a period of about nine months.

If fertilization does not occur, the lining in the uterus is not needed. Within twelve to fourteen days it is shed from the uterus through the process called menstruation. If fertilization occurs, a woman generally does not menstruate again until after the baby is born.

In males, from puberty onward, the testicles, located in the scrotum, produce microscopic cells called sperm. When a man has a sexual climax, called ejaculation, about 300 million sperm are released through his penis. Then the sperm swim into the woman's uterus, where some make their way to the woman's fallopian tubes. If only one sperm comes in contact with the egg, fertilization will occur.

If you suspect you are pregnant, what should you do? It is risky business to try to find out on your own if you are pregnant. Some girls' periods are irregular, and missing a month or two does not necessarily mean they are pregnant. In addition, worry and stress can sometimes cause a girl to skip a period. On the other hand, there have been cases where girls have continued to have their periods while pregnant.

The most accurate way to find out is to have a pregnancy test performed by a professional health care worker. This can be done at a public health clinic, hospital, family planning clinic, abortion clinic, or even a pharmacy. Although home pregnancy test kits are available, they are not 100 percent accurate; they should never be substituted for a laboratory test that shows whether the pregnancy hormone is in your urine or blood, and a pelvic exam by a doctor to check for changes in the size of your uterus.

If you do not want to tell your parents of your suspicions, perhaps you can confide in a close relative, school counselor, or other adult who will help you. If not, there are organizations in every community you can ask for help. One such organization is Planned Parenthood, which is listed in the

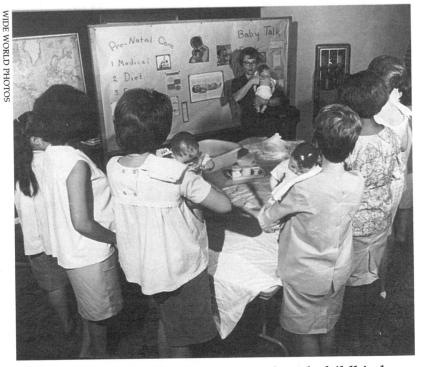

Many cities offer free prenatal and childbirth classes for pregnant teenagers.

White Pages and the Yellow Pages of your telephone directory. This organization offers free pregnancy tests, counseling about alternatives to parenting, including inexpensive or free abortions, assistance in arranging adoptions, and parenting classes. Planned Parenthood absolutely will not contact your parents without your permission.

The United Way and the March of Dimes Foundation can also refer you to people who will help you deal with your pregnancy. Do not be afraid that the people at these agencies will notify your parents or lecture you about why you shouldn't have gotten pregnant. These organizations exist to help pregnant women, not to put them down or judge them in any way.

If you are not considering abortion, you can look up "Maternity Homes" in your telephone directory. These places frequently provide free prenatal care, a place to live and continue your education while pregnant, adoption assistance, and childbirth and parenting classes. A more complete list of people to contact for help with an unplanned pregnancy is provided in the Appendix at the end of this book.

Supporting and nurturing another human being is a big responsibility. It is even harder when you are not yet an adult yourself. While your life from now on, if you decide to keep your baby, will be more difficult than that of teenagers who are not also young mothers, you do have ways to overcome the hardships. Or you may decide that being a parent at this time in your life is not in your best interests. This book provides information about your options so you can make a responsible decision as to what is best for your future and, if you choose to go through with your pregnancy, for the future of your baby.

TWO

Exploring Your Options: Having an Abortion or Keeping Your Baby

ONCE YOU KNOW for certain you are pregnant, you have four options to consider. You can choose to have an abortion, to give your child up for adoption, to marry the father of the baby and jointly raise your child, or to become a single parent. These are weighty decisions that need to be thought out carefully. What you decide will affect many people—you, your parents, the father of the baby and his parents, and of course your baby.

Legally, however, only you and the baby's father have the right to make the final decision about your pregnancy. No one else can force you into any course of action. Therefore, do not let anyone talk you into doing something you feel uncomfortable with. There are advantages and disadvantages to each option. Consider the consequences of each before making a decision.

Patty was fourteen when she became pregnant. "When I told my mom, she said, 'We're getting you an abortion. You're too young to have a baby.' My father was so mad he wouldn't even speak to me. But he agreed with her about the abortion. I told her I wanted to keep my baby, but she made me go with her to this clinic.

"The social worker there asked me how I felt about being pregnant, and I said I didn't want to have an abortion. The lady said it was up to me, that my parents couldn't force me to have it. So my mom took me home. She and my dad were really mad at me for a long time afterward. But I'm still glad I didn't let them talk me into having an abortion. If other girls want to have one, they should. But I just couldn't do it."

Years ago, when a teenager became pregnant, there were fewer options open to her. In most cases, the girl and the father of the baby dropped out of school and got married, usually with the boy getting a low-paying job that did not require a high school diploma; or the girl went away to "live with relatives" for a while. In reality, she was most likely living at what was then called a "home for unwed mothers" until her baby was born, at which time she would give up the infant for adoption and then return home, her secret safe.

Some pregnant girls, however, risked their lives to have illegal "back-alley" abortions. There were uncaring, dishonest men and women who would perform abortions for a few hundred dollars. Because abortion was against the law, women and girls had no medical or legal protection. Usually the abortionists were not doctors or nurses, did not use sterile instruments, and did not perform the abortion in clean surroundings. Often it was done on a dirty kitchen table, and the instrument used was a knitting needle or a wire hanger.

Many girls died from the procedure, either by bleeding

to death or from infections caused by the unclean conditions in which the abortion was performed. Of the girls who survived, many were so ripped up inside that they could not have children in the future. It is a sad fact that even today some girls who do not know about the existence of free or inexpensive legal abortion clinics still resort to back-alley abortions. Other girls try to cause a miscarriage by doing strenuous exercise, taking hot baths, or drinking castor oil. These methods are dangerous, and they seldom work.

After the sexual revolution of the late sixties and early seventies, no longer was it believed that "nice girls don't" have sex before marriage. It became more acceptable to have a child outside of marriage (often called an illegitimate child). Today many unmarried teenagers are choosing to keep their babies. At the same time, however, it is much harder for teenagers to get decent jobs without at least a high school education. Consequently, many teen parents are on welfare of some sort.

You do not have to be a victim of your situation, however, letting early motherhood and possible poverty and unemployment set the course for the rest of your life. You do have alternatives. You may want to talk over your choices with your parents, a close relative, or another adult. If not, you may wish to contact organizations such as Planned Parenthood that offer pregnancy counseling. People at these agencies will listen to your feelings about being pregnant and help you sort out those feelings by talking over the pros and cons of each alternative. They will not try to talk you into doing anything you don't want to do.

While it is a good idea to take your time making a decision, it is unwise to wait too long or to do nothing about your pregnancy. For if you choose to have your baby, you are depriving yourself and your baby of good prenatal care. Many doctors, for example, prescribe special vitamins to provide the nutrients necessary to keep the mother well nourished and to give the baby a healthy start in life.

In addition, a doctor can check to make sure the baby is developing properly, and can handle any complications that might arise. Moreover, if you are considering abortion, time is crucial. For after the eighth week of pregnancy, the risks of major complications or death from an abortion rise with each week you delay.

It is normal for a girl to feel unsure about her options, especially abortion. You may experience mixed emotions of guilt, fear, and grief, both before and after an abortion. That is why organizations such as Planned Parenthood have counselors to help girls deal with these powerful feelings and come to terms with their decisions.

Of the 1.1 million teenagers who become pregnant each year, about 40 percent choose abortion. An estimated 125,000 more would choose abortion if they knew where to go to get one. Most girls have mixed feelings: they do not want to have a baby while they're teenagers, but they do feel a maternal urge to nurture a baby. This conflict makes it hard for them to reach a decision to have an abortion. No decision is 100 percent right. Each alternative will seem wrong to someone. Many girls choose to keep their babies, not because they strongly want to be mothers at the time, but because they cannot accept any other decision.

Abortions performed during the first three months of pregnancy cost less than those performed from the thirteenth to the sixteenth week; after the sixteenth week, the cost goes up still more for each additional week of pregnancy. Some girls do not get abortions because they mistakenly believe they cannot afford them. There are, however, abortion clinics that provide free or inexpensive services.

Moreover, in all states, federal Medicaid funding is available when the woman's life is in danger. In some states, Medicaid will pay for abortions under other circumstances as well. A Planned Parenthood agency or your local Department of Health or Social Services can tell you the laws in your state and how to apply for funds, if available. You may want to ask Directory Assistance for the telephone numbers of these agencies. In addition, the National Abortion Federation has a toll-free hot line that will refer you to a facility in your area. The hot line number is 1–800–772–9100.

If you are considering abortion, you should know that in some states, the law requires that your parents be notified or give their consent before you may obtain an abortion. However, a teenager who feels she cannot tell her parents has the right to appear before a judge, who will determine if the girl is mature enough to make the decision herself. This process is known as judicial bypass. Again, an organization such as Planned Parenthood can tell you about the parental consent laws in your state, and can explain how to initiate judicial bypass.

Abortions are relatively simple procedures if performed during the first three months of pregnancy. The most common method is called vacuum aspiration, and is done in a clinic or hospital. You are given a shot of an anesthetic, similar to the Novocain given by your dentist, to numb your cervix, or you may be sedated with a medication like Demerol or Valium. A clamplike instrument clasps the cervix to keep

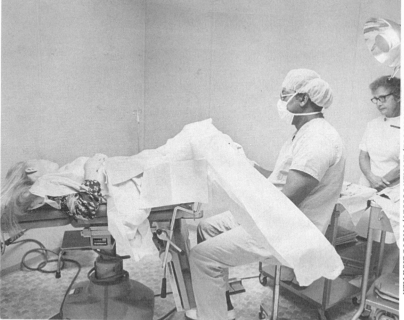

THE ALAN GUTTMACHER INSTITUTE, ESTHER BUBBLY, PHOTOGRAPHER

*During the first three months of pregnancy,
abortions can be performed in a clinic
without an overnight stay.*

the uterus steady. Some women feel only a little discomfort; others feel moderate pressure and some pain.

Next, the doctor widens your cervix by inserting a series of narrow rods (dilators). You may feel some menstrual-type cramping at this point. The stretching takes only a couple of minutes. Then the doctor places a blunt-tipped tube into the uterus through the opening in the cervix. The tube is attached to a small suction machine that removes the fetus. The entire procedure takes about fifteen minutes.

Afterward, you rest in a recovery room until you're ready to leave that same day. You may feel a little weak or tired, and you may experience some cramping. There will be some bleeding as well, about as heavy as a period. Most women recover quickly. You should visit the doctor for a checkup in two to three weeks.

During the fourth month of pregnancy, abortion is a two-step procedure called a D&E, meaning dilation followed by evacuation. Widening of the cervix is performed as in the vacuum aspiration abortion, except that the stretching may be done by inserting very slim rolls of absorbent material that expand gradually. These have to remain in place for several hours. In most cases, you will go home overnight, and then return to the clinic the next day.

In the second step of a D&E abortion, the uterus is emptied through a suction tube and then is cleaned with a curette (a spoon-shaped instrument). When it is over, you spend some time in the recovery room. You should make a checkup visit within two weeks.

In a D&E abortion, there is more risk of bleeding, infection, and incomplete abortion. Your enlarged uterus has thinner walls, and the chance of an instrument poking a hole in the uterus is greater. There is also a slight chance that when the cervical dilators are inserted, the membranes containing the amniotic fluid (bag of water) within the uterus could be broken, and then the second part of the procedure would need to be done right away.

In most places, by about the fifth month, pregnancy termination is no longer done through the vagina. At this stage, you are given a local anesthetic in the skin of the lower abdomen. A needle is inserted through the abdomen into the amniotic sac, which contains the fetus. Some of the amniotic fluid is withdrawn and replaced by a saline solution or prostaglandin. This brings on contractions anywhere from twelve to seventy-two hours later that expel the fetus and placenta through the vagina. The injection method is usually done in a hospital and means staying overnight or longer. The chance of complications is greater than with early abortion or D&E.

In rare cases, the injection method is not successful or cannot be used, and major surgery is performed, called a hysterotomy. This operation is different from a hysterectomy, in which the uterus itself is removed. In a hysterotomy, an incision is made through the abdomen into the uterus, and the fetus and placenta are removed. A hospital stay of five to seven days is necessary, and any children you have in the future may need to be delivered by cesarean section.

After any abortion method, you should be given written instructions for taking care of yourself. These may include taking showers instead of tub baths for a while and using sanitary pads instead of tampons for a few weeks. You may have some bleeding for several days or weeks. Intercourse during that time should be avoided. Your regular menstrual periods usually start again in a month or two.

But remember, *you can get pregnant within two weeks of your abortion.* In addition, you should be aware that having repeated abortions may make it impossible for you to carry a later pregnancy for the full nine months. Therefore, if you do not want to get pregnant again, you should use some form of contraception. You can start using birth control pills right away. At your follow-up visit, the doctor can fit you with a diaphragm. You can use the contraceptive sponge only after all bleeding stops, but you can always use foam or a condom.

The earlier an abortion is performed, the safer it is. As with any kind of surgery, some discomforts and problems may develop, such as upset stomach or cramping. These usually disappear within a few weeks. However, you should call your doctor if they continue. If you experience heavy bleeding, severe adominal pain, or fever, call your doctor immediately. Complications are much less likely to happen if you follow your doctor's instructions for aftercare.

In about one in five hundred cases, abortion fails to end the pregnancy, and the procedure has to be repeated; the second abortion may require hospitalization. This usually happens in mutiple pregnancies (such as twins or triplets) or when the pregnancy is in one of the fallopian tubes (an ectopic pregnancy) instead of the uterus. Ectopic pregnancy is extremely dangerous to the mother, and major surgery is usually performed to remove the pregnancy.

Here is what some girls said about their decision to have an abortion.

Doris was fifteen when she became pregnant. "I just thought, 'How can I take care of a baby? I'm not even old enough to drive a car.' And my folks already had four children to support. I was so young. I wanted to stay in school and go to college and have a career. There was no way I could do both. So I had an abortion.

"It wasn't something I'm proud of, or that I did at the spur of the moment. I mean, it wasn't like choosing what movie to go to or what clothes to wear. I thought about it a lot, and I decided an abortion was best for me. Now I'm a freshman in college, and I take the pill even if I'm not dating anyone special. I never want to go through another abortion. With my next baby, I want to know I want it, and be happy when the doctor tells me I'm pregnant."

Suzanne, sixteen, had intense mixed feelings about her abortion. "Practically as soon as I missed my period, I phoned my boyfriend. He came over, and we talked for hours about what we should do. Finally we decided we were too young to raise a baby. He said he'd go with me to this abortion clinic that one of my friends had gone to. We didn't tell our parents. We were too ashamed and afraid of what they'd say. We both had money saved up from summer jobs, so we used that to pay for it.

"I cried all the way to the clinic, I was so upset. I mean, I didn't want to have an abortion, but I didn't want to have a baby, either. The doctor was real nice. He told me everything he was doing. He gave me a pill to make me sleepy. Then I felt a stick when he gave me a shot to numb my cervix. I had cramps, like the ones I get during my period, when he widened my cervix, and then I heard this low humming noise. That was the suction tube taking out the pregnancy. That was the worst part—knowing the baby, or whatever had developed so far as a baby, was being pulled out of me to become nothing.

"For a long time afterward, I had nightmares where I'd hear that suction noise. I'd wake up screaming. I started seeing a psychiatrist, and I'm glad I did, because now I don't have that dream so often. About the abortion? I don't know. I can't say I'm glad I had the abortion, but I can't say I wish I hadn't had it. What I *can* say is that I wish I hadn't gotten pregnant so young in the first place."

Anita, seventeen, found the decision so difficult that she waited until she was four months pregnant to get an abortion. "I felt so guilty about getting rid of my baby that I could hardly do anything for those four months—eat, sleep, study, even talk on the phone or watch TV or read a book. But finally I knew I just couldn't have the baby. My family was on welfare already, and our apartment was too tiny to add one more person. I told my mother. She was really upset, but she stuck by me through the whole ordeal.

"But I'd waited so long that I had to have a D&E, which is more complicated than abortions done in the first three months you're pregnant. I had to go twice to the clinic— once to get these rolls of material put in to widen my cervix, and again the next day to have the suction tube put in my cervix to take out the baby. It was an awful experience, let me tell you—having to go home and know that my body was getting ready to have my baby taken out of me.

"A couple of my friends had abortions right away, and they didn't go through the depression and guilt for as long as I did. If you want an abortion, get it as soon as you know you're pregnant, or don't get an abortion at all. In fact, if I ever get pregnant again—which I don't think will happen, because I'm on the pill now—I don't think I'd get an abortion. The hurt is just too much."

Eighteen-year-old Anna's mixed feelings caused her to wait even longer than Anita did to decide to have an abortion. "I just couldn't make up my mind, so when I finally decided to get an abortion, I had to have it done in the hospital and stay overnight. The doctor gave me a shot in my stomach where the baby's water sac is, and later that night I started contractions that made the placenta come out, just like having a baby, only there was no baby to have anymore.

"The abortion didn't hurt as much as what happened afterward. They put me on the maternity floor, which meant I heard the babies being brought from the hospital nursery to their mothers to be fed. Every time I heard the babies cry it was like these knives stabbing me in the heart. Once I was standing in the hall when the nurse walked by rolling this big cart with the babies in their plastic cribs. I started crying so hard I thought I'd never stop. I kept thinking I could have been holding a baby like those."

Marla, seventeen, who had her abortion when she was about two months pregnant, had a less agonizing experience. "It wasn't anything I did lightly. It was the hardest decision I've ever made in my life. The doctor gave me a shot, and I sort of went to sleep. Then I woke up, and I had cramps a little, and I was bleeding, like in a period. When I think how my boyfriend told me he didn't want to use a condom because it would take away his pleasure, I get so mad. I wonder how I could have been so dumb to believe a line like that. He got all the pleasure, and I got all the trouble. Don't ever believe boys when they tell you lines like that."

If you do not want an abortion, you may be considering keeping your baby. If so, you are probably thinking about whether you will marry the father or raise your baby alone.

In the fifties and sixties, an "honorable" man was expected to marry the girl if he "got her pregnant," even if he did not love her. Often the girl and her parents saw marriage as the only solution, in order to give the baby a name, meaning the father's last name.

Increasingly, however, teenage girls, and their parents, are discarding marriage as the automatic answer to pregnancy. Many of these girls' parents married early and do not want their daughters to go through the many problems that they faced. Moreover, they know that parenthood will add an extra burden to the marriage.

More teenage girls who want to keep their babies are choosing to raise their children alone. These girls are taking a close look at what kind of relationship they have with the baby's father. If that relationship seems lacking in mutual respect and love, or if the boy does not have a genuine desire to become a father, most pregnant teenage girls decide not to get married.

Jan, who was eighteen at the time her baby was born, says, "At first I thought about marrying my baby's father. He and I were living together anyway. But about a week after I came home from the hospital, he and I started fighting. He would want to go out, and I'd say we couldn't because the baby was so young and I didn't trust a baby-sitter yet. Or he'd want to have sex, but it would be time to feed the baby. He never put the baby's needs first. So after about three months, we split up. Now I'm not tense all the time because of feeling torn between the baby and my boyfriend."

Another girl who decided to become a single parent says, "My boyfriend didn't want to get married. He wanted to let his parents adopt the baby, and he would pretend to be the baby's brother. I told him that wouldn't work. He wanted a baby, but without all the responsibilities. I told him to forget it. I'd raise the baby myself."

Teenagers who choose to become single parents and who are not being helped out financially by their own parents

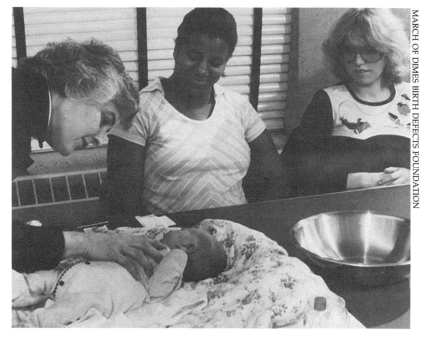

In a child care class, these girls learn how to bathe, feed, and change a baby.

are placing an extra burden on themselves. Most likely they will be going to school, studying, working part time, and taking care of a baby all at once. Trying to fit all that into twenty-four hours each day has caused many teenage parents to give up one of their responsibilities, most often school. By doing so, they become stranded in low-income jobs, receiving welfare to supplement their income.

There are, however, resources at your disposal. A family planning clinic or a local Planned Parenthood organization can help you become part of a teen parent program. This organization can also show you how to apply for financial assistance through Medicaid, which finances health care for pregnant adolescents and adolescent parents, or through Aid to Families with Dependent Children (AFDC). If one resource does not provide the help you need, whether financial, emotional, or vocational, the clinic or Planned Parenthood can direct you to an organization that does.

Marriage can either ease or add to the burden of parenting, depending on the kind of relationship you have with the father of the baby. If he is a responsible person, is employed, and has an enthusiastic and supportive attitude about the baby, your marriage has a better chance of succeeding, and caring for your child will become easier, since you will not carry the full responsibility of raising your baby alone.

The statistics on teenage marriages are not encouraging, however. Almost half end in divorce. Studies also show that half of the teenage mothers who marry become pregnant again within the next three years. This means the chances are good that a girl will be a divorced single parent raising more than one child. As one girl says, "I thought taking care of one baby was hard. But raising two babies is almost impossible. When one gets sick, the other gets sick. And it's really hard to watch your two-year-old and give your baby a bottle at the same time."

Getting married for the sake of the baby seldom works, and getting a divorce is more difficlut when a child is involved. "My folks kept telling me to get married, but I said no," a fifteen-year-old girl remembers. "Pregnancy isn't a good reason to get married. And I knew my boyfriend and I couldn't afford to raise a baby. If we got married, our parents would have said, 'You've got to keep the baby. You're married now.' "

Exploring Your Options

Of course, many teenage marriages do succeed. But it takes an enormous amount of hard work. Joan's story is an example. "Don and I have been married for over a year now, and we're making it. He works as a mechanic during the day and goes to night school. I go to a teen mother school that has a day care center for our daughter, Jenny. In the afternoons I leave her at another day care center while I work as a checker at a supermarket. I'll graduate from high school this June, and then I'll go to nursing school, so eventually I can support us while Don goes to college."

Joan has obviously done some careful planning for herself and her family. She also has the support of her husband in making their marriage work. Other couples, like Bob and Lilah, live with one of their parents while they finish school.

"It's hard to feel like a mother when you live with your own mother," Lilah says. "Mom still treats me like a kid, even though I have my own kid now. But Bob and I are trying to get along with my folks, because they're really helping us out by letting us live with them, and we want to make a happy home for our son. Sometimes we argue about how bossy my parents are, but we made a rule that we'll talk about whatever's bugging us, even if we have to stay up all night to settle an argument."

Bob and Lilah's marriage has a better chance of succeeding because they are committed to their relationship and their child. Her parents will help them financially and emotionally through the difficulties of raising a child while still in their teens.

As a single or married parent, you will be responsible for your baby twenty-four hours a day every day of the year. This may not sound like much while you are pregnant and can generally decide what you want to do and when you want to do it. After your baby is born, however, you will not be in complete control of your free time. If, for example, you suddenly feel like taking a walk or going shopping at three o'clock in the afternoon, that might be the moment when your baby needs feeding. Therefore, you won't be able to drop everything and walk out the door. And anytime you want to go out alone, you will have to find a sitter.

Many teenage parents find being tied down this way extremely frustrating and often depressing. As one single teenage mother says, "I thought you could just call up a sitter service and that was it. I didn't realize all that went into having sitters—like making sure they know when to feed the baby and what to feed her. And making sure I look up the phone number of wherever I'm going to be in case of an emergency."

Another single mother adds, "And even when I do go out, I can't have as much fun as I did before, because I'm always worried that something might happen to the baby while I'm gone."

The feeling of being tied down can undermine a marriage as well. This is what it was like for Margie and her husband:

"Chuck and I thought it wouldn't be any problem to get married and raise a baby. We had so much fun dating that we thought marriage would be even better. We didn't count on not having any extra money to go out with our friends. All our own money and the extra money my folks gave us went for the baby and paying the bills. We also thought our folks would baby-sit anytime we wanted to go out. No way. They said, 'This is your baby, and you're responsible for it.' "

Another married teenage mother says, "When we didn't have a baby to take care of, we thought we were rich from the salaries we made from our after-school jobs. We never realized how much it costs to live decently, to feed a baby, and to pay the doctor when the baby is sick. Things were so tense between us when our little boy got sick that we nearly got divorced. I didn't know how to take care of a well baby, much less a sick one. I really love Andy, but if I had it to do over again, I don't know . . . I just don't know."

Many teenage mothers share this disillusionment with parenting once they actually start caring for a baby. One girl says, "I thought having a baby would make me feel grown up. It was just the opposite. I couldn't do anything right with the baby, and I felt helpless."

Another teenage mother confesses, "My folks and I didn't get along, and I thought having a baby would get me away from them and solve all my problems. I'd have someone who really loved me. Well, I got someone who really loves me, all right. But my problems aren't anywhere near solved. If anything, I've got more problems now than ever before—trying to hold down a job and go to school and take care of my daughter all at the same time."

Before considering marriage, it might be a good idea to ask your boyfriend how much help he plans to give in taking care of the baby and how he feels about becoming a father. Does he have a job? Will his or your parents be able to help out financially? Will you both be able to stay in

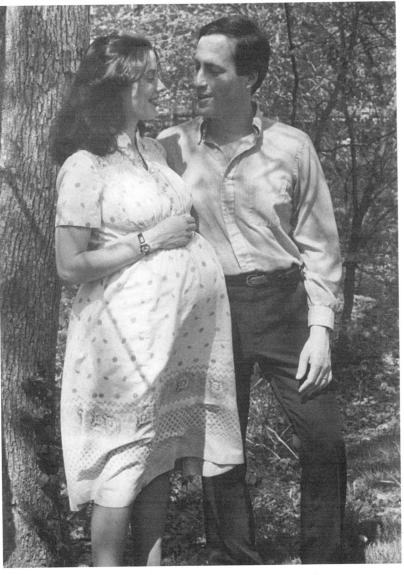

Traditionally, raising children has been a two-parent job.

school if you marry? Will you have a decent place to live?

Even if you can answer yes to all these questions, you will find that maintaining a good marriage takes work. And working on having a good marriage at the same time you are learning how to become a good parent may be too big a job.

Heather, a single teenage mom, says, "People told me it would be hard raising a kid all by myself. Trouble is, I didn't believe them. Even if I had, I wouldn't have known how hard it really is. Try to imagine having to feed a baby every four hours for twenty-four hours a day. No time off for sleep, either. And babies have to be changed a lot, and they cry whenever they want anything. Believe me, that crying can drive you crazy. I love my son, but I wouldn't advise anybody to try what I'm doing. When your baby needs something, there's nobody around to say, 'Oh, let me do that for you.' It's all on your shoulders."

Sixteen-year-old Susan has this to say about parenting: "Nobody told me how many times a day you have to change a baby's diaper, or that you have to sterilize the bottles and heat the formula just right so it won't be too hot. And I thought all babies did was eat and sleep. Uh-uh. They cry a lot. Sometimes even if you rock them, feed them, and change them, they still don't stop crying. I kept thinking it must be my fault. I'm doing something wrong. No. Crying's just part of what babies do."

In addition, many girls do not stop to think that babies grow up. When children begin to crawl and then to walk, they want to touch and explore their environment. No longer is a child content to just eat and sleep. Now he or she is awake most of the day and needs attention every minute of that time.

Toddlers do not know the difference between dangerous sharp objects and soft cushiony ones. They will put anything they can find into their mouths. Therefore, all medicines, insecticides, cleaning fluids, and other poisonous substances must be kept well out of their reach. Cabinets, closets, and areas behind televisions or other furniture are potential danger zones for the toddler. Electrical outlets and cords are a particular hazard, as toddlers will stick things into the sockets. Mothers cannot leave their children alone for one second, for fear they will hurt themselves.

Keeping track of your children becomes more time-consuming as they grow older. One young mother explains, "When Timmy started kindergarten, I thought, 'Whew! He's finally on his own.' Wrong. Now he wants to be taken to other kids' houses to play, or to the park, or anywhere I go. And I have to take him to school and pick him up every day even if I'm sick."

"Now I know why they call two-year-olds the 'terrible twos,' another teenage mother says. "Kelley won't do anything I say. It's always no! to whatever I ask her to do. Bedtime is a real hassle. She's constantly asking for one more story or one more glass of water."

After reading these girls' stories, you can probably understand why raising children has traditionally been a two-parent job. Most of the time, it takes two people to make the difficult job less burdensome. When a mother and father raise their child together, one parent can take over when the other is sick, overly tired, or simply too frustrated to perform the job successfully. In other words, a mother and father raising a child together can give each other rest periods, which all parents need, no matter how easy their children are to handle.

Although recently there has been a decline in the number of two-parent families, the ideal time to have children is after you are married and when you are financially and emotionally capable of raising children. For practical and emotional reasons, parenting is easier when it is a shared experience. And sharing that experience usually makes it more rewarding.

Whether you are married or single, however, before

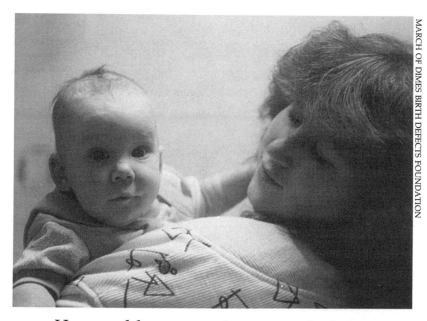

MARCH OF DIMES BIRTH DEFECTS FOUNDATION

Hugs and love are as important for babies
as teaching and discipline.

you choose to keep your baby, take an honest inventory of what you can give your child and what he or she can give to you. If you find that your list of what the baby can give you is very long, it is likely that you will be disappointed in motherhood. Because babies are helpless and demanding, they need to be taken care of constantly, and they do not always give you back the warm cuddly response you expect.

Raising children can also be a rewarding, happy experience, however. Parents who calmly set limits on their children's behavior, while expressing love and a genuine respect for their children, generally have an easier time. Children are natural mimics. If they see their parents screaming and out of control, they will copy that behavior.

Classes and books on child care can be a great help to young parents. But most experts in child care agree that the main ingredient for successful parenting is love. Touching, holding, hugging, and kissing are as important as teaching and disciplining. There was good sense behind the bumper sticker that said, "Have you hugged your child today?"

THREE

The Adoption Option

IF YOU DO NOT WANT to get an abortion and you do not want to become a parent, adoption might be the right option for you. Adoption is a legal process by which permanent legal custody is transferred from the birth parents to other parents. Some girls hesitate to choose adoption because they mistakenly believe the adoptive parents will not love their child or care for it properly. The truth is that there are far more people wanting to adopt babies than there are babies to be adopted. While only about twenty thousand babies a year are put up for adoption, there are two million couples wanting to adopt—averaging out to approximately eighty couples who want every infant available for adoption. Therefore, if an adoption agency places your baby, only the best qualified parents will have a chance to adopt him or her.

Adoptions may be arranged in three ways. In a private adoption, you may place your baby with any person you choose, subject to the approval of the courts. Thus, you know where your child is and with whom he or she is living.

The second method is the independent adoption, in which the child's placement is arranged by a third person, such as a lawyer or doctor.

In both private and independent placements, it is wise to keep in mind that people with little training in child placement may be involved in deciding the future of your child. A much less thorough investigation of the adoptive parents will be done, and they usually receive no counseling. In fact, in independent adoptions, anyone who can afford the price can adopt your child. You will have little or no choice about who adopts your child, nor will you have information about them. Moreover, if problems arise, the adoptive couple can give the child back to the person who arranged the adoption or to the courts at any time, even years later.

This is not true in the third method of adoption, the agency placement, in which a state-licensed adoption agency makes all the arrangements. These arrangements include adoption counseling and most or all of the prenatal care and hospital costs for the birth mother, a thorough screening of the people who apply to the agency to adopt a child, and required adoption counseling for the prospective adoptive parents.

Some agencies are affiliated with state-licensed maternity homes where you can live and go to school until your baby is born. Two of the largest such maternity homes in the United States are St. Anne's Maternity Home in Los Angeles, California, and the Edna Gladney Home in Fort Worth, Texas. At these homes, girls are required to attend the home's high school, counseling sessions, and classes in prenatal care, childbirth, and parenting.

Every state has its own laws for each of these three

methods of adoption, so procedures vary. For example, in eight states—Connecticut, Delaware, Massachusetts, Michigan, Minnesota, North Dakota, Rhode Island, and Virginia— only adoptions arranged by agencies are legal. In all states, if the mother knows the father of the baby, she must name him in any adoption papers she signs. If a married adolescent chooses to place her child for adoption, the law requires that her husband consent to the adoption.

If the girl is unmarried, most states require that the father of the child be notified of any adoption plan and that, if the mother gives up her rights to the child, he be given the opportunity to petition the court for custody of the child. He may be awarded custody if he can prove to the judge that he is able to support and love the child. If the father does not want custody, he is asked to sign an affidavit (a legal paper) giving his approval for the adoption. After the affidavit is signed, the father may not change his mind and try to stop the adoption.

If the father cannot be notified, or if he refuses to acknowledge paternity and signs a paper stating his refusal, then the birth mother retains all legal rights to her child. If you do not know where the father is, you may be allowed to sign an affidavit stating this fact, as long as a reasonable attempt has been made to locate the father. The judge may then declare that the father is not entitled to any notification.

In agency adoptions, you may tell your adoption counselor the type of couple you would like to raise your child. Perhaps you would prefer that your child live in a small town, for instance, or that there be other children in the adoptive family. If you wish, you may also specify the nationality and religion of the couple, or you may request adoptive parents who share your interests and talents. Both birth parents and adoptive parents may know non-identifying information about each other, such as nationality, race, medical history, education, interests, talents, physical characteristics, religion, the adoptive parents' reasons for choosing to adopt, the birth mother's reasons for placing her child for adoption, and information about relatives of both families.

Names and addresses of both sets of parents are kept confidential. Often, however, the adoption agency will let you see photographs and background information on three prospective adoptive couples, and then allow you to choose which couple you want to raise your child.

In most states, after the adoption is final, information about the identities of the birth and adoptive parents is sealed by the courts to protect the privacy of everyone involved. The only way for an adopted child to have the records opened is to petition the court and prove that unsealing the records is necessary because of a medical emergency. Some states have registries at the Bureau of Vital Statistics, located in the state capital, where birth parents and adopted children can register their willingness to meet when the child is eighteen. At that time, a meeting between the birth parents and the child is arranged by state officials.

Other states allow an adopted adult to request a meeting with his or her birth parents, either through the courts or through the agency that handled the adoption. The birth parents are then asked, by a state official or the adoption agency, if they will consent to such a meeting. If they agree, a meeting will be set up. In independent adoptions, the adopted child would have to make such a request through the courts.

You may also leave a letter in your child's file at the adoption agency requesting that you be contacted if your child ever asks to meet you. In addition, you may write a letter to your baby explaining your reasons for placing him or her for adoption, or send a gift, and sometimes even a photograph of yourself, for the adoptive parents to give your child when he or she is older. Agencies encourage adoptive parents to share this information with their children early in life, so that the children know that their birth parents loved them even though they could not raise them.

Moreover, while the child is growing up, some birth mothers and adoptive parents correspond with each other through letters sent to the adoption agency. This allows the birth mother to keep up with her child's progress, and it allows the adoptive parents to know about any medical problems the birth mother might develop.

Some agencies will assist in direct, or open, adoptions, in which the birth mother and adoptive parents meet each other. Open adoptions may include arrangements in which the adoptive parents are present for the birth of the baby. And the birth mother may present the child to the adoptive parents afterward. Continuing communication through the exchange of letters, photographs, gifts, and occasional visits with the adopted child may be arranged. In some cases, regularly scheduled visits are set up.

There are some questions to be considered about open adoption. First, how will you feel about having an ongoing relationship with your child but no right to make decisions about any aspect of your child's life? Second, will the development of the child's close relationship with the adoptive parents be hampered by your continued contact with him or her? On the other hand, in this kind of adoption the birth mother can be certain that her child is all right, and the child's questions about the mother can be answered. This should relieve any feelings of rejection a child may have in knowing he or she is adopted.

What about costs? Placing your baby for adoption is free to you. Most private agencies use the adoptive parents' fees to cover the hospital costs for the birth of your baby. In independent adoptions, all allowable costs incurred by you are paid by the parents who adopt your child. However, if you change your mind and decide to keep your baby, you may have to pay back all or part of that money.

In thinking about couples who want to adopt a child, you might be interested in the costs to them. These include their application to adopt, adoptive counseling, a home study of their qualifications to adopt, supervision by the adoption agency for a trial period after the baby is placed with them, lawyers' fees for completing the legal work involved, hospital fees for the birth of the baby, and possible maternity home care for you. Costs can total over ten thousand dollars. In 1985, according to the National Committee for Adoption, the average cost of adopting a child through a private adoption agency was six thousand dollars.

Parents who apply to an agency to adopt a child go through a thorough screening process. A social worker asks questions about every aspect of their lives, including why they want to adopt and how they feel about raising an adopted child instead of a child of their own. It is an emotionally draining process for the adoptive parents, but the close scrutiny ensures that your baby will be placed with loving, capable people.

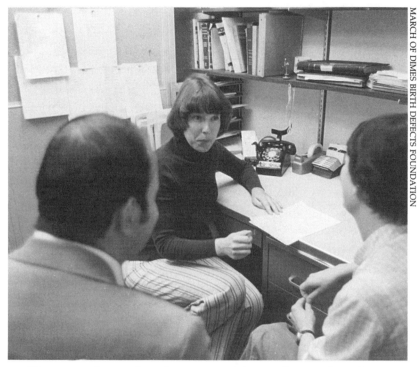

Prospective adoptive parents go through a long screening process before they can adopt a child.

Many agencies have requirements for couples who want to adopt a child. These requirements may include an age limit—between twenty-five and forty-five, for example. Agencies may also require that the couple undergo a complete medical examination; that they have been married for at least three years; that they can afford to support a child; and that one of them will stay at home with the child for the first year or two.

If the agency accepts the couple, they are put on a

waiting list. Agency social workers try to match them with the requests of the birth mother as to who should adopt her child, and, using the background information they have about the birth mother, try to decide which of all the adoptive parents on their list will be the most compatible parents for a particular child.

After the adoptive parents are chosen, they take the baby home and file a petition to adopt the child. This is only the first step in the legal process of adoption. The next step is a trial period of one to six months, during which time the agency's screening process continues. The adoptive parents' social worker visits them regularly to make sure the child is being well taken care of and loved. If, after the trial period, the agency believes that this couple is capable of raising the child, the adoptive parents petition the court to make the adoption final. If the court approves, a final adoption decree is issued. At this time, the child becomes a legal member of the adoptive family, with all the rights of any child born to the family. The child is given the family's last name, and an amended birth certificate is issued naming the adoptive parents as the child's legal parents.

If you decide to place your child for adoption through an agency, you will not sign any legal papers giving up your child (relinquishment papers) until *after* the birth of your baby. In fact, even in private and independent adoptions, you cannot be held legally responsible for signing relinquishment papers *before* your baby is born. You may sign these papers in the hospital, but usually you will be asked to wait at least seventy-two hours after giving birth to assure the court that you are no longer under the influence of any medication you might have received during the delivery of your baby. In some states, you must sign the papers before a judge.

You may also decide whether or not you want to see your baby. *No one can deny you this right.* Some girls choose not to see their babies at all, feeling that any contact with their child might make it impossible for them to go through with the adoption plans. If you do want to see your baby, you may hold him or her and take photographs as well.

You also have the right to name your baby on the original birth certificate, although once the adoption is final, the adoptive parents may change the name. The name they choose will go on the amended birth certificate and become the legal name of your child. Your name and address will not appear on the amended birth certificate.

If you place your baby with an agency and do not use an open adoption method, you will not know the new name of your child, and your child will not know his or her original name, as the original birth certificate will be sealed along with the adoption records. Neither will the adoptive parents know your name or address. In all states except Kansas and Alabama—where the original birth certificate is available to any party to the adoption, including the adopted child when he or she becomes eighteen—the only way to open these records is to show a "just need" to the courts.

If, after your baby is born, you are still unsure whether adoption is right for you, adoption agencies will place your baby with a foster family until you make up your mind. However, the earlier you decide on adoption, the better chance your child will have for a placement. This is because the majority of adoptive parents want to adopt infants rather than older children.

Do not sign any legal papers until you are sure. Once you sign those papers, you cannot change your mind and have your baby back. In agency placements, the adopting couple will not be notified that they have been accepted as adoptive parents for your baby until after you sign the relinquishment papers, even if you have picked the couple out yourself.

Placing your baby for adoption may very well be the most painful, wrenching decision you will ever make in your life. In this situation it is normal for you to have mixed feelings of guilt, relief, and grief—the same grief, perhaps, that you would feel if someone very close to you died. The difference is that your baby did not die. It is only the feelings that are the same. You may wonder whether placing your baby for adoption was the right choice. You will probably think about your baby often and wonder how he or she is doing, especially on your baby's birthday. For a while after you place your baby, you may feel lonely and depressed.

One advantage of an agency placement is that your adoption counselor will continue to be available to you for as long as necessary after the adoption is final. You should never hesitate to ask your counselor for a meeting to talk over your feelings and any concerns you have about your decision or your child's well-being. In addition, some agencies have support groups for birth parents, in which you may share your feelings with other teenagers who have gone through the adoption experience. Most girls say talking about their feelings with others in their position helps to relieve their doubts about their decision and makes them feel better emotionally.

How do mothers make this very painful decision to give up their babies for adoption? Some mothers say that

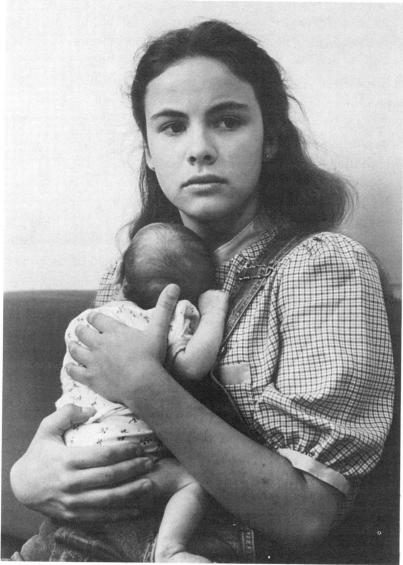

Whether or not to place a baby for adoption is a difficult, painful decision that takes a lot of thought.

they try to take an honest look at their ability to care for a child, both financially and emotionally. They think about their goals for themselves and for their baby, then ask themselves if they can accomplish those goals while raising a child. Or they take a realistic look at what they can offer their child in the areas of education, time, and special needs. For example, can they give their child a chance to grow up in a two-parent home with mature, responsible people? After thinking about these questions, the birth mother may decide that people who are already married and established in careers, who want a baby but who cannot have one, would be the best parents for their baby.

Sharon, age fifteen, says, "I thought adoption would be best for my baby. I wouldn't have to go on welfare, and I figured parents who had good jobs and couldn't have babies of their own could give my little girl more than I could."

Cindy, who also chose adoption, says, "I told my boyfriend, 'What else can we do? I'm fifteen, and you're sixteen. We fight all the time, so if we got married we'd probably get divorced, and even if we didn't, we don't have jobs, we haven't even finished high school, and we don't even know what we want to do with our lives, so how could we take care of a baby?' I just wasn't mentally ready to take care of a child. I knew I had to get myself together before I could take care of someone else."

Another girl, who was not completely happy about the idea of adoption, nevertheless chose that option because, as she says, "I was fourteen, and couldn't get a job, since you have to be sixteen to get most jobs. So there was no way I could take care of him. Plus I was only in the eighth grade. Somehow, being a mother in the eighth grade just didn't seem like it was old enough. Even so, it's really sad after you do it, because you don't realize how much you love your baby until after you give it up."

Sally was only thirteen when she became pregnant. "When I was pregnant, all my friends were going to parties and to the beach and having fun, while I was stuck at home because I didn't like going out and having everybody stare at me. But I didn't like not hanging around with my friends. I thought, 'Well, if this is how you feel now, when the baby isn't even born yet, think how you'll feel when you really have to say home and take care of a baby.' It wouldn't have been fair to keep my baby and feel that way."

After going through the adoption experience, many girls say they felt very relieved and very sad at the same time. One girl says, "I was crying all the time I was pregnant, trying to decide what to do. After he was born, I kept thinking, 'I want to keep him, but what kind of life can I give him?' For the next year, lots of times I would just start crying, I still felt so bad about giving him up. But I signed a paper at the adoption agency saying if my son ever wants to find me, they should give him my name and address. Because I'll always consider him my son, no matter what."

Another girl explains, "The part about adoption that I really worried about was whether my baby would hate me for giving her up. So I wrote a letter to her for the adoptive parents to give her. I told her how much I loved her, and that it was because I loved her so much that I gave her up, because I could never have given her everything I would have wanted to."

And another says, "When the social worker asked me about giving my baby up, I was shocked. I thought, 'How could a mother do such a thing?' But then she told me how there's waiting lists a mile long of people who want to adopt babies, and that only the best qualified parents get to adopt. So then I thought, 'I could love my baby easy, but these other parents can give her all the things I can't right now.' It's been two years since the adoption became final, and I still think of her every day. But when the social worker tells me that she is such a happy, healthy baby, I know I did the best thing for her by giving her up."

"The only way I could give my baby up for adoption was not to see her at all," says Margaret, seventeen. "I was adopted myself, and my adoptive parents picked me up straight from the hospital the day after I was born. I wanted it to be like my adoption. I also knew if I saw her it would make things a lot harder. I'd probably have freaked out and wanted to keep her. So when she was born, I kept my eyes closed while I pushed, and kept them closed until they took her out of the delivery room. Now that I've coped with it, though, I want to get pictures to see what she looks like. A lot of people tell me I shouldn't see pictures, but I think it will fill that little gap in the back of my mind.

"Later, this nurse at the hospital told me she had gotten pregnant while she was married and given up her baby because she and her husband couldn't afford to take care of a child then. That made me feel better to think that here was this lady who *was* married, and still she gave up her baby. At the time, she was going to nursing school, and, like me, didn't want help from her parents to take care of a baby. Now she and her husband earn a good living. And they have five kids."

For Natalie, sixteen, giving her baby up for adoption

was a difficult emotional experience, the pain of which stayed with her for a long time afterward. "I don't think you ever forget," she says. "I keep thinking, 'How old will he be when I'm twenty-five, or thirty?' Every time I see a happy mother pushing her baby around in a stroller, I feel sad. I wonder, 'Is that my baby?' I look at the mother and at the baby to see if they look alike."

Nineteen-year-old Amy's frame of mind about her decision to place her baby can be considered ideal. "It's been almost a year now, and I'm still sure I made the right decision. It was the hardest one of my life, but adoption was the only choice that made sense to me. I was a senior in high school, and I had no way of supporting a baby. I had five brothers and sisters, so I knew my parents couldn't take on another child. But I got to pick out my baby's parents from three choices. I know their first names, that the father is an attorney, and that the mother is a real-estate agent who paints for a hobby. So do I.

"When I held my baby for the last time in the hospital, it was almost impossible to let her go. I thought I'd never stop crying, and I wanted to change my mind. I still cry when I think about it. But at least I know she's loved and taken care of by two very nice people. And there's always a chance she'll want to know me when she's eighteen. I left my name and address with the adoption agency just in case. Yes, it hurt like crazy to give my baby up, but it was the only choice—for both of us. There will always be a part of her in me. After you carry a baby inside you for nine months, signing a piece of paper doesn't take away your baby's place in your heart. Never."

F O U R

The Next Nine Months:
Prenatal Care for
You and Your Baby

T HE NEXT NINE MONTHS will probably be the most crucial, in terms of health, in your life. Everything that you take into your body—by eating, drinking, or inhaling—your baby also will take into his or her body. That is why it is important to get good prenatal care. This means taking care of yourself, and thus your baby, while you are pregnant, which will help increase your chances of having a healthy baby.

Many pregnant teenagers, however, delay getting medical care and advice or receive no prenatal care at all, sometimes because they do not want anyone to know they are pregnant, or because they fear that they cannot afford to see a doctor. Today many teen pregnancy programs provide free or inexpensive medical care, as well as classes on nutrition, exercise, and childbirth, continuing education, vocational training, food assistance, and day care facilities after the baby is born. You may also be eligible for Medicaid or another assistance program.

Your local family planning clinic, Planned Parenthood

center, or March of Dimes chapter can tell you how to apply for federal aid. Moreover, some of these organizations sponsor group meetings in which pregnant adolescents talk about prenatal care and their feelings about being pregnant. In addition, you may be eligible for health insurance coverage provided by your employer, if you have a job, or through your boyfriend's or parents' employee medical insurance plans. Your school nurse or counselor may also know about programs for pregnant or parenting teenagers.

For instance, the WIC program (Special Supplemental Food Program for Women, Infants, and Children) provides food for eligible pregnant women and the babies they later deliver. Food stamps are also available for eligible teenagers in most areas. Ask at your doctor's office or your local city or county health department about these two programs. (For health department telephone numbers, look in your telephone directory or ask Directory Assistance.)

Because so many teenagers do not get prenatal care, the statistics on the health of babies born to teenage mothers are not encouraging. Teenage mothers are at greater risk of having babies with birth defects, mental retardation, breathing difficulties, or epilepsy. Nearly twice as many infants born to mothers age seventeen or under die within the first year of life, compared to infants born to mothers age twenty or over. In addition, teenage mothers are three times more likely than older mothers to have low birth-weight babies (less than 5.5 pounds). Low birth weight is associated with infant death as well as serious childhood diseases, brain defects, and mental retardation.

Teenage mothers themselves are more likely than mothers over twenty to have complications resulting from premature births and to develop toxemia and anemia. For mothers under age fifteen, the death rate from pregnancy complications is also higher than it is for older mothers.

Children born to teenage mothers are less able to handle stress than are children of older mothers; they score lower on intelligence tests; and they are more likely to have to repeat a grade in school, have behavior problems, and be on a lower reading level than children born to adult parents.

You will have a better chance of rising above these statistics if you get good prenatal care. The first step in having

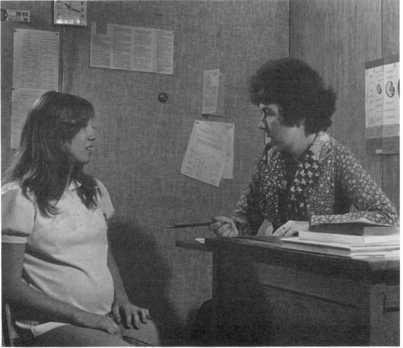

Good prenatal care includes seeing your obstetrician regularly.

a healthy pregnancy and a healthy baby is to see the obstetrician who will deliver your baby. An obstetrician is a doctor specializing in women's reproductive health, including care of a woman during pregnancy, labor, and delivery. The obstetrician will be able to answer all your questions about pregnancy and instruct you on good nutrition, exercise, and care of yourself throughout your pregnancy.

You can help prevent problems by making regular visits to your obstetrician during the entire nine months. These visits usually are scheduled once a month for the first six months, and then every two weeks until your ninth month, when your doctor will want to see you every week. Make a list of questions you have and take it with you to your appointment. Your doctor will also ask you questions about your periods, any previous pregnancy, any medical problems in your family, whether you use birth control, and if you have had any problems with your birth control method. It is important for you to answer completely and honestly. Be sure to mention any medicine you were, or are, taking.

At each appointment, you will be weighed and your blood pressure will be taken. At your first appointment, samples of urine and blood will be taken to check if you have diabetes, anemia, the Rh-negative blood factor, or a kidney or bladder infection. Later on, the size of your pelvis and the growth, position, and heartbeat of your baby will be checked. In addition, the doctor will examine your eyes, ears, nose, throat, thyroid, chest, breasts, and abdomen.

The obstetrician will also perform a pelvic examination to check the size, shape, and position of your uterus; this will help tell how far along your pregnancy is. You might feel nervous about a pelvic exam if you have never had one; most people feel some anxiety when they do not know what to expect. Perhaps you'll feel better knowing that a pelvic examination does not hurt and lasts only a few minutes. Some girls worry that the exam will reveal facts about their sexual life. For instance, they think the doctor can tell how often they have had sex. This is not true. The purpose of the exam is to determine whether your reproductive organs are healthy.

For at least twenty-four hours before the exam, do not douche or use any vaginal preparations that could cover up some vaginal conditions. (Many doctors recommend not using these products at all, especially when you are pregnant.) You will feel more comfortable if you urinate just before the exam.

When you go into the examining room, you will be given a robe or a sheet to cover your lower abdomen and thighs so you will feel less exposed. Pelvic examining tables have metal stirrups. You lie on your back and rest your heels in these stirrups after sliding your hips down to the edge of the table. To relax your body and make the exam less uncomfortable, breathe slowly and deeply with your mouth open; let your stomach muscles go soft; relax your shoulders and the muscles between your legs; and ask the doctor to tell you what is being done during each step of the exam.

The pelvic exam involves three parts: the speculum exam, the bimanual exam, and the rectovaginal exam. First, in the speculum exam, the doctor checks the vulva and vagina for redness, irritation, discharge, cysts, or other conditions that may need attention. The doctor then inserts an instrument called a speculum into the vagina to hold the walls

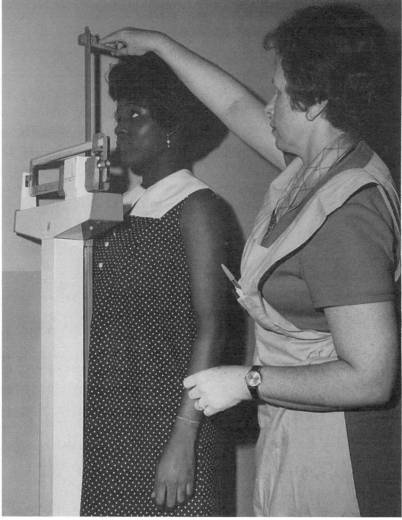

Each time you see the doctor during your pregnancy, you will be weighed to make sure you are gaining the amount of weight needed for your baby's development.

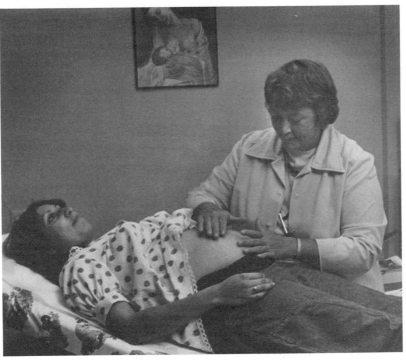

*An obstetrician feels the position of the baby
during a prenatal examination.*

of the vagina apart so that he or she will be able to see the cervix and vaginal walls. You may feel some pressure or a cold object, if the speculum is made of metal. The doctor checks for any growths or abnormal discharge from the cervix. Tests for gonorrhea and chlamydia may be taken by collecting cervical mucus on cotton swabs.

Next a Pap smear is taken by inserting a cotton swab and a small wooden or plastic spatula, which looks like a tongue depressor, inside the vagina. Cells are gently collected from the cervix, and the "smear" is sent to a laboratory for examination. The Pap smear is used to detect pre-cancerous or cancerous cell changes and to identify cells indicating herpes, yeast, or other infections. At this time, the vaginal walls are checked for irritation, injury, or other abnormalities.

The second step of the pelvic exam is the bimanual exam, in which the doctor feels your internal organs. He or she will be looking for any tenderness or pain, which might indicate infection; the size, shape, and position of the uterus; any abnormal growths; any swelling of the fallopian tubes; any enlarged ovaries, cysts, or tumors. In the bimanual exam, the doctor inserts one or two gloved, lubricated fingers into the vagina. The other hand is used to press down on the lower abdomen to feel the internal organs of the pelvis. You may feel a bit uncomfortable. Deep breathing with the mouth open helps. You should feel no pain, but if you do, tell your doctor.

There may be a third part of the pelvic exam. This is the rectovaginal exam, in which the doctor inserts a gloved finger into the rectum to check for possible tumors located behind the uterus, in the lower wall of the vagina, or in the rectum. You may feel you need to have a bowel movement during the procedure, but this is normal and lasts only a few minutes.

The description of a pelvic examination sounds as if it takes a long time. The actual time is not more than ten minutes, usually less. Do not be afraid to express your concerns about your pregnancy and delivery, and to ask the doctor any questions you want, even if the question is not about pregnancy.

It's exciting to look ahead and imagine the changes that

will take place during the coming months. Pregnancy is often divided into three periods called trimesters. Each is about three months long.

THE FIRST TRIMESTER

During the first trimester, you will probably find it hard to believe you are pregnant. Most women gain only three to four pounds. Your baby grows to three inches long and develops all of his or her major organs. You may experience some nausea in the morning.

Your First Month

For the first eight weeks, the baby is called an embryo. The heart, lungs, and brain are beginning to develop, and the heart will beat by the twenty-fifth day. The embryo is enclosed in a sac of fluid to protect it from bumps and pressure. The umbilical cord also develops at this time. The cord is made up of blood vessels, which carry nourishment from your body to feed the baby, and the baby's wastes back into your blood to be eliminated.

Your Second Month

Arms, with tiny hands and fingers, and legs, with the beginnings of knees, ankles, and toes, are starting to form. The stomach and liver have also begun to develop. The head seems very large compared to the rest of the body, because the brain is growing so fast. Tiny ears and the beginnings of hair are forming. You may tire more easily and need to urinate more frequently now.

The Next Nine Months

Your Third Month

The embryo is now a fetus, which means "young one." It is about three inches long and weighs about one ounce. Signs of the baby's sex are beginning to appear. Fingernails and toenails develop, and the mouth opens and closes. The baby moves its hands, legs, and head, although you cannot feel this movement. Your clothes should begin to feel tight. You may also feel warmer than usual.

THE SECOND TRIMESTER

In the second trimester, most of the morning sickness you felt during the first three months of pregnancy disappear, and you feel especially good. You can feel the baby move, and you will start to look pregnant.

Your Fourth Month

Your baby weighs about six ounces and is about eight to ten inches long. You should gain three to four pounds and start to "show." You may feel a slight sensation of movement in your lower abdomen, like bubbles or fluttering. If you write down the date you first feel this movement, called "quickening," your doctor can better determine when your baby is due.

Your Fifth Month

Your baby weighs about a pound and is about twelve inches long. The doctor can hear the baby's heartbeat, and you can feel more definite movements. You may gain three or four pounds and begin to breathe deeper and more frequently. The area around your nipples may look darker and wider as your breasts prepare to make milk.

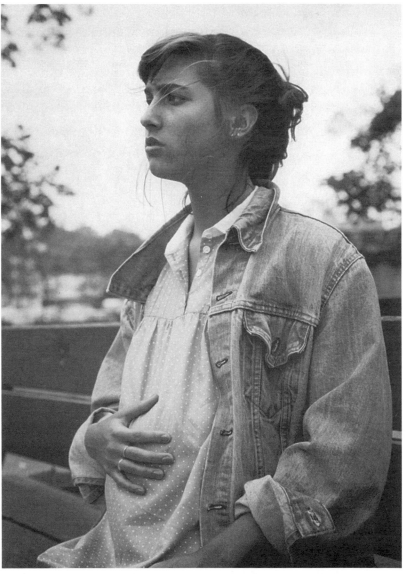

During the fifth month of pregnancy,
mothers can feel their babies move.

The Next Nine Months

Your Sixth Month

You are now carrying a fully formed miniature baby—about 1½ pounds and fourteen inches long. Its skin is wrinkled and red, and there is practically no fat under the skin. The baby sucks its thumb and goes through the motions of crying, without making a sound, as its vocal cords are not fully formed. You will feel the baby move regularly. You may gain three or four more pounds and experience some backache.

THE THIRD TRIMESTER

As your baby grows larger, you may experience some discomfort from pressure on your stomach or bladder. You will feel the baby's stronger and more frequent movements.

Your Seventh Month

Your baby is about fifteen inches long and weighs about 2 or 2½ pounds. The baby exercises by kicking, stretching, and changing positions from side to side. You may be able to see the movement when one of the tiny heels or fists pokes you. You may gain another three or four pounds and notice some slight swelling in your ankles.

Your Eighth Month

Your baby has grown to about sixteen inches long and weighs about four pounds. Its eyes are open, and it moves to a new position in the uterus. This position is maintained until the baby is born. You may gain three to five pounds.

Your Ninth Month

At thirty-six weeks, your baby is about nineteen inches long and weighs about six pounds. The baby's weight gain now is about one-half pound per week. At forty weeks, your baby is "full-term" and usually weighs from six to nine pounds. Your baby settles farther down into your pelvis, and people will say your baby has "dropped." This is called "lightening." Your breathing will be easier, although you may need to urinate more frequently.

There are several myths about pregnancy that you should know are *not* true. A common one is that if you look at something ugly or frightening, your baby will be deformed. Nothing you look at will deform your baby, and conversely, listening to classical music will not make your baby artistic or smart.

Other ideas that are *not* true are that reaching over your head will make the umbilical cord strangle your baby or that eating certain foods, such as strawberries, grapes, or blueberries, will give your baby birthmarks. The truth is nothing you eat causes birthmarks. They are caused by an abnormal distribution of melanin or an abnormal condition of the blood vessels in the skin. Whenever you hear something about being pregnant that sounds odd or scary, ask your parents, doctor, nurse, or counselor whether it is true. More than likely it is not.

At the beginning of your pregnancy, after you have seen your obstetrician, the next step in good prenatal care is healthy nutrition. The higher death rate for children born to teenagers is more closely related to inadequate nutrition and prenatal care than to the age of the mother. Even if you are overweight when you become pregnant, this is not a time to diet. Do not take diet pills, and do not skip meals.

Normally, you should gain between twenty to thirty pounds during the entire nine months. If you are underweight, you may need to gain more than that amount. Usually pregnant women gain about one pound a month for the first three months. From the fourth month on, it is best to gain at least three to four pounds a month. Your doctor will tell you how much weight gain is right for you. You probably will return to your normal weight about three months after your baby is born. If you breast-feed, you may return to your pre-pregnancy weight sooner, since breast-feeding will help use up the fat your body stored during pregnancy.

What you eat affects your baby's health. Your baby develops within a fluid-filled sac in the uterus. The amniotic fluid in this sac keeps the walls of the uterus from hampering the movements of the developing fetus. It also protects the fetus from heat and cold and acts as a shock absorber if you fall or get hit in the stomach. A new organ, called the placenta, forms on the wall of the uterus. It is connected to the navel of the fetus by an umbilical cord that looks like a rope of jelly. The placenta carries food and oxygen from your blood to the fetus through this cord. The fetus's wastes return the same way to your bloodstream. Your kidneys get rid of the baby's wastes along with your own.

Almost everything you take into your body crosses over to the fetus. That is why alcohol, cigarettes, and drugs affect your baby's development. Women who smoke are more likely to have low birth weight babies, and smoking during breast-feeding will pass the nicotine on to the baby. Babies born to smoking mothers have a higher incidence of sudden infant death syndrome (crib death); they are more susceptible to respiratory problems, and they may be slightly behind their age group in physical growth.

Many people do not realize that alcohol is a drug. It depresses the central nervous system and affects nearly every organ in your body. When you take a drink, the alcohol crosses through the placenta into the fetus. Then it travels through the baby's bloodstream. So when you take a drink, your baby takes a drink. Women who drink even one ounce (the amount of alcohol found in two standard drinks) or less of alcohol a day while pregnant have a greater chance of miscarriage, stillbirth, or delivering premature, physically deformed, or mentally retarded babies.

A significant number of infants born to women who drink heavily during pregnancy have such serious physical, mental, and behavioral abnormalities that these babies are said to have been born with "fetal alcohol syndrome" (FAS). Babies with FAS are shorter, weigh less than normal, and do not catch up with healthy babies, even after special postnatal care is provided. FAS babies also have abnormally small heads, facial irregularities, joint and limb abnormalities, heart defects, and poor coordination. Most are mentally retarded, and many are hyperactive, extremely nervous, and have short attention spans.

You should also be aware that many cough medicines and nightime cold remedies contain large amounts of alcohol. If you breast-feed, the alcohol from these medicines and from drinks will pass to your baby through your breast milk in the same concentration as it is in your blood.

Today, with the incidence of drug abuse so high, doctors

are especially concerned about the effects of drugs on unborn babies. Drugs taken by a woman during pregnancy pass through the placenta into the baby. Therefore, if you are hooked on drugs, your baby will be an addict, too. Addicted babies are born in excruciating pain because they are going through withdrawal from the drugs the mother has taken. Many of these babies die. The ones who survive often have physical defects. A tragic example occurred during the late 1950s and early 1960s when women in Germany and England were using the drug thalidomide, a supposedly safe sedative sold without a prescription. Thousands of infants were born with deformed limbs or no limbs at all.

Prescription and over-the-counter drugs should be used only with the approval of your doctor. Even the prescription hormones estrogen and progestin, found in oral contraceptives, if used during the first three or four months of pregnancy, can increase the risk of birth defects. Therefore, women who become pregnant while using oral contraceptives should stop taking them immediately and consult their doctor. Women who stop taking the pill in the hope of becoming pregnant should use another form of contraception, such as a diaphragm or vaginal gel, for at least three months before attempting to conceive a child.

Other drugs associated with birth defects are amphetamines and antibiotics such as tetracycline, which causes permanent discoloration of the baby's teeth. Barbiturates taken in the last three months of pregnancy increase the chance of delivering a baby addicted to barbiturates. Tranquilizers such as Valium increase the risk that the baby will be born with a cleft lip or palate. Even aspirin can cause serious side effects and definitely should not be taken during the last three months of pregnancy, except under a doctor's supervision. Aspirin contains salicylate, which may prolong pregnancy and labor and cause excessive bleeding before and after delivery.

While it is true that pregnant women experience periods of anxiety and stress, there are better ways to handle these feelings than taking drugs or alcohol. First you might ask yourself just what is bothering you, and if there is any specific action you can take to improve the situation. Or you might try talking over your feelings with someone close to you. At other times a long walk or listening to music might help relieve your tension. If you think you may have an alcohol or drug problem, you can find help by phoning your local affiliate of the National Council on Alcoholism, Alcoholics Anonymous, or other such self-help groups.

In addition, X rays and other medical radiation procedures should be avoided during pregnancy. X rays of your abdomen, stomach, pelvis, lower back, or kidneys may expose your unborn baby to the X-ray beam, which can cause changes in your baby's cells, which are dividing and growing into special cells and tissue. Any change in this cellular process can cause birth defects or illnesses such as leukemia later in life. This is another reason why you should not keep your pregnancy a secret from your doctor.

Now that you know what *not* to take into your body while you're pregnant, what *should* you eat and drink to keep yourself and your baby healthy?

Eating well nutritionally will help ensure that your baby gains the right amount of weight before it is born. When you are pregnant, you need about 300 more calories each day than you normally do. You can get these extra calories

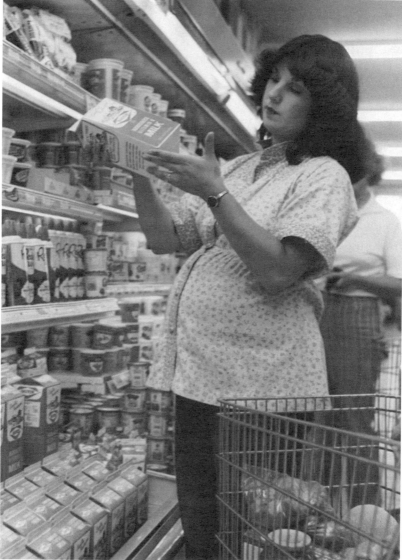

*Good nutrition is vitally important for
your health and that of your baby.*

by eating larger amounts of some of the foods you eat often. For example, one extra half glass of milk and an extra half sandwich each day will give you those additional 300 calories. When you are breast-feeding your baby, you will need 500 more calories a day than you needed before you became pregnant. Milk is an important source of calories, protein, and calcium for mothers who breast-feed.

You should eat foods from all four food groups every day. Fruits and vegetables give your body the vitamins, minerals, carbohydrates, and fiber necessary for growth and energy. You will need to eat four servings of fruits and vegetables every day. A serving is about one-half cup, or the amount typically eaten at one time—for example, one apple or half a grapefruit.

Out of these four fruit and vegetable servings, you need at least one serving that contains vitamin A, such as apricots, broccoli, carrots, dark green leafy vegetables, or watermelon; and one serving that has vitamin C, such as cabbage, grapefruit, orange juice, or green peppers.

Breads and cereals give you minerals and vitamins. Whole-grain breads and cereals give you fiber to prevent constipation. You should eat five or six servings of whole-grain bread or cereal every day while pregnant and while breast-feeding. Be sure to use margarine on your bread and unsaturated oil in your salads or in cooking. You should also have one-half cup of rice or corn, or a potato, or three tortillas each day.

Milk and dairy products give you the extra protein, calcium, and other nutrients you need while pregnant. Each day you need to drink four or five eight-ounce glasses of milk. If you cannot drink milk, ask your doctor how to get calcium from other foods. Make sure your milk says "Vitamin D Added" on the label. When judging the amount of milk you drink, remember to include the milk in other foods such as milk shakes, cream soups and sauces, macaroni dishes, puddings, custards, cereals, and yogurt.

Meat, fish, chicken, turkey, eggs, dried beans, peas, seeds, nuts, and peanut butter supply protein and minerals such as iron and zinc. You need three or more servings of these foods daily to get enough protein while you are pregnant and when you breast-feed. If you are a vegetarian, you will need to discuss food choices with your doctor.

Try to avoid fried foods, as they are hard to digest. While snack foods, desserts, candy, and soft drinks supply calories, they do not supply enough of the nutrients you need. If you fill up on these foods, you may not eat the foods you really need. Some foods from this group, however, although high in calories, also have important amounts of other nutrients. Such foods are sweet potato pie, pumpkin pie, custard pie, carrot cake, banana bread, bread pudding, rice pudding, and oatmeal, raisin, and peanut butter cookies.

You should also drink six to eight glasses of water or other liquids each day. Women who breast-feed their babies need eight to twelve glasses of liquid a day. However, tea, coffee, cocoa, chocolate, and many soft drinks have caffeine in them, which is not good for an unborn baby. If you drink these liquids, choose decaffeinated brands.

You will probably feel more comfortable during the last three months of your pregnancy if you do not eat a lot of food at one time. You may want to eat several small meals instead. If your doctor says you are not gaining enough weight, try eating extra servings of bread, cereal, milk, or protein foods. If you get a lot of exercise, you will need more than 300 extra calories a day.

Besides eating well, you need to get plenty of rest— eight hours of sleep each night and a fifteen-minute rest once or twice a day. You also need exercise while you are pregnant. Exercise will help you feel and look better and will aid in digestion and circulation. In addition, exercise often makes for an easier labor and delivery. Ask your doctor what kinds of exercise are safe for you. Generally, walking, dancing, bicycling, and swimming are exercises you can do safely while pregnant. There are also special exercises that can help you in labor and delivery. These are taught in prenatal classes. Ask your doctor about these classes and about childbirth preparation classes in your area.

You can generally continue working until the sixth or seventh month. How long you will work after that depends upon how you feel and what your doctor advises. It is also safe to have sexual intercourse while you're pregnant. Your doctor may ask you to abstain from sex during the last three or four weeks before delivery, however. It is also normal for your feelings about sex to change during this time. You may experience periods when your desire for sex increases or decreases. See your doctor as soon as possible if intercourse is painful or if you have any bleeding.

Avoid lifting heavy objects and moving furniture while you are pregnant. Stretching will not harm you or your baby, but do not reach for things while standing on a chair or ladder, because you might lose your balance and fall. During the last months of your pregnancy, you will probably feel awkward because your balance will be affected by your increasing size.

There are also some annoying, though not serious, side effects of pregnancy. Morning sickness is an example. This is nausea and vomiting that usually occurs in the first three months of pregnancy, often when you first wake up in the morning. Eating a few soda crackers or dry toast when you first wake up may help control nausea. Try leaving some soda crackers beside your bed before you go to sleep at night; when you wake up, eat the crackers before you get out of bed. Stay in bed a few extra minutes without moving. Then get up slowly. Instead of drinking liquids with your meals, wait an hour or more before drinking anything.

A frequent need to urinate is another bothersome side effect of pregnancy. This occurs because the growing baby is pressing on your bladder. If you have a burning or itching sensation when urinating, tell your doctor. As your baby grows larger and takes up more room, you may become short of breath. This problem will go away close to the time your baby is born. Moving more slowly will help.

Constipation is also common during pregnancy, as the muscles in your intestines become more relaxed. In the last months of pregnancy, the growing baby puts pressure on the lower intestines, which may also cause constipation. Exercising; eating whole-grain breads, cereals, raw fibrous fruits, and vegetables; and drinking plenty of liquids will help to prevent constipation. Never use laxatives, enemas, or any home remedies without first checking with your doctor. Constipation and straining may lead to hemorrhoids. Tell your doctor if you have painful or bleeding hemorrhoids.

You may get heartburn while pregnant. This has nothing to do with your heart; it is a burning feeling that usually comes after eating; it occurs because the baby is pushing against your stomach. To avoid heartburn, try to relax, chew your food well, and eat slowly. Instead of eating three large meals a day, eat several small meals. Cutting down on spicy and greasy foods can also help.

Varicose (enlarged) veins might appear in your lower legs. These are caused by your enlarged uterus, which presses on your abdominal veins and interferes with the return of blood from your legs. Varicose veins usually shrink or disappear during the first few weeks after the baby is born. You can help avoid varicose veins by not wearing tight stockings or socks. Do not stand in one place for long periods of time, and don't sit with your legs crossed. Sit with your feet propped up whenever you can. Support hose may also help prevent varicose veins.

Leg cramps may occur in the last months of your pregnancy; they are also due to pressure from your enlarged uterus. These cramps frequently occur when you are in bed. A heating pad, a massage, or stretching the calf muscle may bring relief.

You may have a thick white discharge from the vagina. Do not use tampons while you are pregnant. This discharge is a sign of infection if it is bloody, yellowish, greenish, or dark, or if it has a bad odor or causes burning and itching. Tell your doctor immediately if these characteristics are present in your discharge. You can help prevent vaginal infections by bathing daily, wearing cotton undergarments, and avoiding tight slacks or pantyhose.

Skin changes, such as splotches or brownish spots on your face, or dark or reddish streaks on your abdomen and breasts, may appear. These "stretch marks" are due to the stretching of your skin; they generally fade after pregnancy.

The Next Nine Months

You have probably heard women talk about craving certain foods during pregnancy, such as ice cream, strawberries, or pickles. If you crave any of these foods, it is all right to eat them in moderation. Some women even crave nonfoods such as dirt, ice, starch, baking soda, or clay. This type of craving is thought to be the result of inadequate iron in the mother's diet. If you experience such non-food cravings, do not eat these non-foods. Instead, tell your doctor.

During the first three months of pregnancy, your emotions go through many changes. You may feel happy one day and sad the next. Some days you may be very irritable, and others very calm. During the last months of pregnancy, you may feel uncomfortable, unattractive, and nervous, and you may have trouble sleeping. Some days you may feel weepy and grouchy, and on other days you'll feel happy and excited. All pregnant women go through these mood changes.

It is even common for the father of the baby to experience mood changes during your pregnancy. At times he may feel helpless and left out, and at other times he may be overly concerned about his new responsibilities. Fathers-to-be often feel more included in the pregnancy if they go with the mother to the doctor and to childbirth classes, and if they are with her during labor and delivery.

If you take care of yourself, you should have a healthy pregnancy. However, sometimes problems do develop. For instance, you will have blood tests during pregnancy to see if you are anemic, which means you do not have enough red blood cells. Red blood cells are important because they carry oxygen needed by you and your baby. The most common cause of anemia is not eating enough foods high in iron. Pregnant teenagers need extra iron. Your doctor will probably tell you to take iron tablets and folacin (a vitamin that helps protect the body against anemia) during pregnancy. The best way to prevent anemia is to eat foods like liver, red meats, dried beans, leafy green vegetables, and fortified cereals. Try to avoid drinking tea with your food, because tea prevents your body from using most of the iron found in foods.

Another serious complication of pregnancy is toxemia, which is also called pregnancy induced hypertension, or PIH. Toxemia is high blood pressure, along with protein in the urine, or water retention, or both. Toxemia can progress to convulsions in you and your baby. PIH, if it is going to occur, usually happens after the twentieth week of pregnancy. Tell your doctor immediately of any sudden weight gain, swelling of the feet and hands, severe headaches, dizziness, blurred vision, or spots before your eyes. PIH can usually be successfully treated if diagnosed early.

If you notice bleeding from your vagina and severe stomach cramps, call your doctor immediately. Save the pads you wear to catch the blood, because the doctor will want to inspect them. This bleeding and cramps could be the sign of miscarriage—when the fetus is born before it has developed enough to live outside the mother's body. In some cases, miscarriage is nature's way of preventing the birth of a baby who could not have survived. Miscarriages can usually not be prevented.

Another cause for concern is if you have what is called the negative Rh factor. Your blood will be checked for a substance called the Rh factor. If your blood contains this

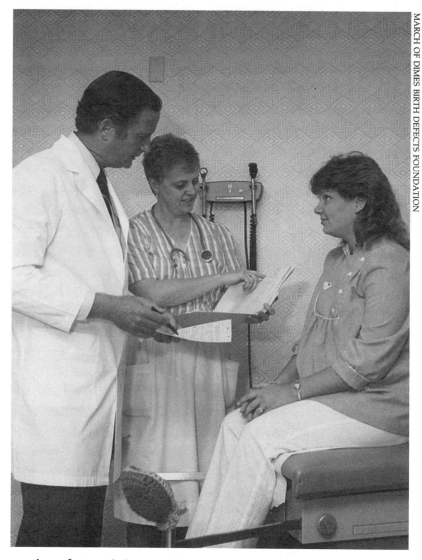

An obstetrician and a nurse go over this young woman's progress during her pregnancy and answer her questions.

factor, you are Rh positive. If not, you are Rh negative. If you are Rh negative and the baby's father is Rh positive, there is a possibility that your baby's blood may also be Rh positive, the opposite of yours. In this case your body manufactures substances called Rh antibodies that will affect your unborn baby's Rh positive blood cells.

Antibodies are normally useful, because they protect you from many common diseases. In this case, however, the antibodies can make your baby anemic. The Rh factor does not usually affect your first baby. However, you will have to receive an injection of Rh immunoglobulin within seventy-two hours of every delivery, miscarriage, or abortion to protect each baby in future pregnancies.

There are other possible complications that require a doctor's attention immediately. Phone your doctor if you are exposed to venereal disease, German measles, or hepatitis. Also phone right away if you have severe or continuing nausea and vomiting; sharp or continuous pain in the abdomen; chills and fever; unusual rashes or sores on the skin; dizzy spells or fainting; or a sudden gush of water from the vagina before the scheduled delivery date of your baby.

To feel more comfortable during pregnancy, wear loose clothing and a bra that fits well. If your breasts are large, you may want to wear a bra at night, too. About the middle of pregnancy, your nipples may drip a small amount of clear or yellowish fluid, called colostrum. This is a sign that your body is preparing for breast-feeding. Colostrum can dry into a crust around your nipples. It should be washed off only with warm water, since soap dries out the skin and makes your breasts sore. If colostrum is heavy, wear a cotton or absorbent pad in your bra. Be sure to replace the pad often.

Wearing low-heeled shoes during pregnancy helps your posture and takes the strain off your back and legs. After the fifth month, as you become heavier, you may get cramps in the muscles of your legs or abdomen. Lying down with your feet up often helps. Avoid standing or sitting for long periods of time. In addition, many women perspire more during pregnancy because their bodies are going through many hormonal changes. Bathing and washing your hair often will make you feel more comfortable. Never douche during pregnancy unless your doctor tells you to.

You may feel a bit overwhelmed by all the do's and don'ts of pregnancy. Yet behind all the advice is an important truth: *What you do does make a difference.* As Dr. Walter H. Glinsmann, chief of the Federal Drug Administration's clinical nutrition branch, said, "Getting pregnant is like running a race. You have to get yourself in condition."

FIVE

Labor and Delivery

Aᶠᵗᵉʳ ɴɪɴᴇ ᴍᴏɴᴛʜs of being pregnant, wondering whether your baby will be a boy or a girl, and who he or she will look like, you are probably more than ready to have your baby and find out the answers to these questions. If you are like most pregnant women, you are probably also a little nervous about the birth of your baby. What will labor be like? Will it hurt? Will you be able to go through with natural childbirth, or will you choose some type of anesthesia? Although every woman's labor is different, one aspect of having a baby is the same for all women. Giving birth ranks as one of the most, if not the most, thrilling experiences of their lives.

Does childbirth have to be painful? As with any unknown experience, if you have no preparation, or no idea of what is going to happen, the experience can be quite frightening and painful. That is why it is a good idea to take some sort of childbirth preparation class.

In Lamaze classes, you will learn exactly what is happening to your body and to your baby during birth, so that

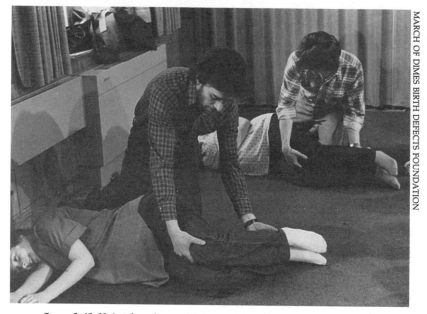

MARCH OF DIMES BIRTH DEFECTS FOUNDATION

In childbirth classes, couples learn breathing exercises that will make labor easier.

the experience will not be frightening. You will also learn breathing exercises to help you relax during each contraction, and pushing techniques to help you push your baby down the birth canal and out into the world. Then you will be more in control of yourself, which makes anyone feel more secure and less panicked.

In addition, if you take Lamaze or other childbirth classes, you may ask someone to take them with you so that he or she can coach you in the breathing exercises and give you encouragement and support during your actual labor and delivery. This person might be your boyfriend, husband, parent, sister, brother, friend, or one of the child-

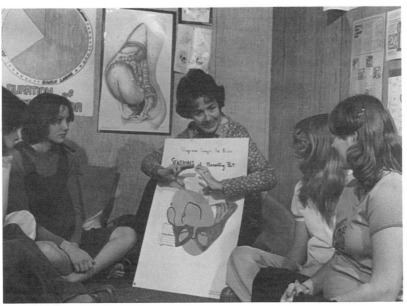

In their childbirth class, these girls learn how a baby progresses through the birth canal during labor.

birth instructors. Most women who learn these breathing and muscle relaxation techniques do not need any anesthetic or painkillers during labor and delivery, and their babies are usually born less wrinkled and red, and more alert.

Sixteen-year-old Jill describes her labor and delivery this way: "Seeing my baby being born was the most exciting experience of my life. I don't think anything else can match it. I won't say the contractions weren't painful, but my boyfriend was my coach, and he really helped me keep doing the breathing exercises, instead of just lying there screaming or crying or something, when the pains got hard. It's amazing how doing that breathing takes your mind off the pain. He kept telling me, 'You can do it. Don't give up. You can do it.' I did, too, and am I ever glad!''

And Kim, who was fifteen at the time, says, "When the contractions got really bad, I asked the nurses for something to knock me out, but my coach kept massaging my stomach and telling me how I was helping my baby be born, and that in just a little while I'd see my baby. That helped me keep going. When I saw my baby actually come out of me, I'll tell you, I started crying. I was so glad I hadn't made them knock me out, because I would have missed seeing her being born. That was worth all the pain.''

Judy, seventeen, remembers her labor and delivery as "the hardest work I ever did in my life. Right before they took me into the delivery room, my contractions were coming so strong I didn't think I could stand it. As soon as one contraction would end, I could feel another one starting. But my coach helped me do the panting breathing so it wouldn't hurt so much. Then my water broke. It was like a big gush whooshed out, and I felt so warm. A nurse examined me, and when she said, 'You're ready. We're taking you into the delivery room,' I was so excited I knew I could get through the rest of the delivery.

"In the delivery room, they put me on this table with my feet in these stirrups and a sheet over my stomach. There was a mirror over my head, and they angled it so I could see everything that was happening. It wasn't embarrassing, because your body doesn't look like it usually does. What you see is this big, dark hole.

"My contractions weren't so bad then, and I had this feeling like I wanted to go to the bathroom. The doctor told me to push, and all of a sudden the baby's head came out.

Everybody in the delivery room was excited. The nurse said, 'Look! There's your baby's head!' And the doctor said, 'Push one more time. Don't shut your eyes. Here comes your baby.' And then I saw her just sort of slide out.

"The doctor held her up, and she let out a howl. It was the sweetest sound I ever heard. I was laughing and crying all at the same time. When the doctor put her on my stomach while he cut the cord, it was the warmest feeling I've ever had, and I thought, 'I love this baby. I love her so much.' "

To be able to see your child take its first breath of air is truly awesome. It boggles the mind to think about how your child started out as a fertilized egg no bigger than the dot over an "i," and within approximately 280 days, or nine and one-third months, grew into the baby lying in your arms on the delivery table.

What should you do to prepare for giving birth? About two weeks before your delivery date, pack a bag with the personal items you want to take to the hospital. These items can include a bathrobe, nightgown (opening in front if you plan to breast-feed), two bras (nursing bras if you plan to breast-feed), underpants, sanitary pads and belt (you will have bleeding similar to having a period for three to four weeks after giving birth), toothbrush, toothpaste, comb, brush, cosmetics, and something to wear home (either maternity clothes or other loose fitting clothes, as you will not yet be back to your pre-pregnancy weight).

If you are keeping your baby, you will also need clothes to take your baby home in. If the weather is cold, the baby will need a blanket, sweater, and cap. If it is warm outside, only a diaper and receiving blanket will be necessary.

You might also want to take some things to make you feel better during labor: a hot water bottle for backache, an icebag for cramps and aches, lotion for massaging your abdomen, chapstick for your lips if they become dry from breathing through your mouth, a breath freshener, and lollipops or sour candy to moisten your mouth.

Plan ahead of time how you will get to the hospital at any time of the day and night. Put telephone numbers in a handy place so that you can call the people who need to be notified when you go into labor. Your doctor is the first person to call, as he or she can tell you if it is really time to go to the hospital. Women often have false labor—contractions of the uterus that do not actually open the cervix. Contractions that are irregular, or that go away when you walk around are a sign of false labor; in real labor the contractions will get stronger.

There are three signs that real labor has begun. One is regular contractions, which usually begin in your lower back and then travel to the front of your abdomen. Contractions occur because your uterus is tightening and relaxing to help open the cervix (the opening at the bottom of your uterus) and push the baby out through your birth canal (vagina). These early contractions may feel like menstrual cramps. They usually come fifteen to twenty minutes apart and last for thirty to forty-five seconds. *Do not eat anything once labor has begun.* In case you need to have anesthetic for a cesarean section, an empty stomach will guard against your vomiting and choking while asleep.

The second sign that real labor has begun is a pink plug of mucus that comes out of your vagina. This is called the "show," and it is caused by your baby pushing against your cervix, which causes the cervix to begin opening. There is also a small amount of blood in the show.

The third sign is a gush or trickle of water from your vagina, which tells you the membrane, or bag of water, that surrounds your baby during pregnancy has been broken. This does not hurt, but feels like a flow of warm water. Your water can break either at the beginning or at the end of the first stage of labor. Call your doctor immediately if your water breaks while you are still at home. If your water does not break, phone your doctor when your contractions are coming regularly fifteen minutes apart. For a first baby, mothers usually come to the hospital when their contractions are five minutes apart. Do not worry that you may not make it in time. The first stage of labor is usually eight to twelve hours long for a first baby.

When you arrive at the hospital, go to the admitting office. Your doctor has probably phoned ahead to tell the labor room nurses to expect you. You will be asked about health insurance and other medical information for the hospital's records. You will then be taken to the labor room, where you will put on a hospital gown. The hair around your vagina may be shaved so the skin will be clean, and you may be given an enema to clean out your lower bowel and rectum. This makes more room for the baby to be born. A doctor or nurse will keep checking you while your labor progresses.

You will feel more relaxed if you concentrate on what is really happening inside you while you are in labor. Your uterus is a muscle that is able to open up to let your baby out through the cervix during birth. Muscles of the uterus pull up on the cervix, first thinning it out, and then opening it up all the way to the size of your baby's head. A contraction is like a great wave—it starts out slowly, builds up to a peak, and then eases off, after which there is a rest period.

There are three phases of labor before you push your baby out: early, active, and transition. In early labor, called *effacement,* your contractions are little waves, and you hardly know you are having them. These contractions, which thin out your cervix, last thirty to sixty seconds, and are between twenty and five minutes apart. You may feel as if you have the flu or as if you are having menstrual cramps. This phase lasts from six to eight hours with your first baby.

In the second phase of labor, called *active labor,* your contractions last from forty-five to sixty seconds, and are from five to three minutes apart. These contractions are dilating, or opening, the cervix to the size of your baby's head. How far the cervix has opened is measured in centimeters. Thus the nurse checking you might say, "You are five centimeters dilated." You will experience more pain in your back, hips, and legs. You may notice an increase in the discharge of mucus. Toward the end of active labor, you may doubt your ability to cope with the contractions, but if you keep doing your breathing and relaxing exercises, the pain will be less severe.

The third part of labor is called the *transition stage.* Until now, your contractions have been opening the cervix. Now they start helping to push your baby down into your pelvic area. Your contractions in this stage of labor are the strongest and most uncomfortable, lasting from sixty to ninety seconds, with only thirty to sixty seconds in between. This will be the hardest part of your labor. Transition may take from twenty minutes to one hour.

During transition, some women feel a loss of control;

they become restless or even panicky and ready to give up. This is the time your coach can give you the most encouragement. Keep picturing your baby moving closer and closer to the opening in your cervix, and keep telling yourself that soon you will see your baby. If you have taken childbirth classes, remind yourself that using the breathing exercises and relaxation techniques you learned will mean a shorter labor, less pain, and more oxygen for your baby. You may feel a great need to push down, similar to the feeling of having a bowel movement. Try not to push unless your doctor or nurse tells you to.

When the cervix is completely dilated, you are ready to push your baby through the birth canal. You will be moved from the labor room to the delivery room, where you will be placed on a delivery table with rests for your arms and stirrups for your feet and legs. Your vaginal area will be washed, and a drape will be placed over your legs and abdomen. There will probably be a large mirror overhead that can be tilted so that you can watch your baby being born.

Now your contractions become less intense, lasting about sixty seconds, with one to three minutes in between. You will feel a lot of pressure in your rectum. This is the *expulsion* phase of labor. Now your doctor or nurse will tell you to push down as if you were having a bowel movement. This usually feels good, relieves pain, and shortens labor. You will experience renewed energy as you see your baby's head emerge.

Your doctor may make a small cut, called an episiotomy, between the vagina and the anus, widening the opening to allow your baby to be delivered without tearing your vaginal tissues. Many women say they never even feel the

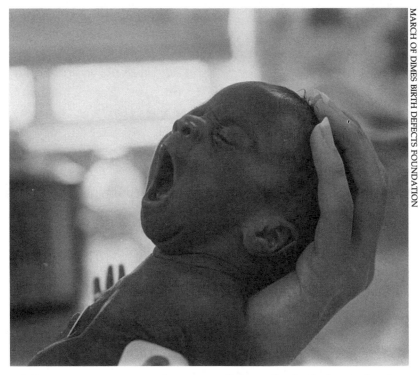

Most women say that watching their baby take its first breath is worth any pain they felt during labor.

episiotomy because they are concentrating so hard on seeing their baby being born. At this time, if your water has not already broken, it will, causing a gush of fluid from the vagina. Once your baby's head is out, pushing with the next few contractions will bring your baby into the world.

At this moment, many women say they experience a feeling of overwhelming happiness. The doctor will hold your baby with its head lowered, in order to drain amniotic fluid, mucus, and blood from the baby's nostrils. A small bulb syringe may be used to clear the baby's mouth and nose. The doctor may place the baby on your stomach while he or she puts drops into its eyes to prevent infection, and then cuts the umbilical cord halfway between the placenta and the baby. Then, if you like, you may hold your baby for the first time.

Keep in mind that your baby has lived in a bag of water for nine months, and has just made a long, difficult trip through the birth canal. Therefore, he or she will probably look red and wrinkled, perhaps with a big head, and with a white, creamy substance all over the body. Nurses will clean this substance off your baby; soon the wrinkles will disappear, and the infant's head will develop the correct shape within a week or so. Your baby will most likely be crying hard when it is born, in order to get air in and out of its lungs. An identification band will be placed on your baby's wrist before leaving the delivery room, and his or her hand- and footprints may also be taken.

The moment your baby is born, your uterus will suddenly shrink and release the placenta from the uterine wall. During the next five to thirty minutes, your uterus continues to contract (this does not hurt) until the placenta and membranes pass out of the vagina. If you had an episiotomy, the doctor will repair it with stitches. The stitches will be absorbed and therefore will not need to be removed. Sometimes an injection is given to numb the vagina area so that you will not feel the stitches.

You will now be taken to a recovery room for an hour or two, where you will be watched closely and checked for any excessive bleeding or unusual change in blood pressure. The baby's father or another support person may be allowed in the recovery room with you. Later you will be moved to your room. Most women stay in the hospital from two to four days.

Many hospitals allow you to have your baby in the room with you so that you can feed, hold, and change your own baby. Hospitals have different policies about whether anyone else may be in the room with you when your baby is there.

You may choose instead to have your baby placed in the nursery. If so, your baby will be brought to you for feeding approximately every four hours during the day if you are not nursing, and around the clock if you are breast-feeding. However, if you are placing your baby for adoption and do not wish to see him or her, just ask your doctor to leave your instructions with the nursery staff.

Babies quickly learn to recognize the voice and the touch of the person who cares for them. Their vision clears fast. Therefore, if you are caring for your baby, remember that babies who are talked to and cuddled are much more relaxed and happy. If you are unsure about how to hold, feed, burp, or change your baby, ask one of the nurses to show you. If baby-care classes are offered by the hospital, ask all the questions you want. No question is foolish.

After delivery, you will be very tired and will probably sleep a lot. You will be encouraged to get out of bed and walk the first day, however. It is important to empty your bladder within six to eight hours after you have your baby. You will probably have a little difficulty urinating, and the nurse can suggest ways to help. If you have extreme diffi-culty, a catheter (plastic tube) may be inserted into your bladder to empty the urine.

Sometimes women have their babies through cesarean section, or C-section. A cesarean is an operation in which the baby is removed through an incision in the abdomen rather than being delivered through the vagina. The operation is performed only under certain conditions, such as when the baby is in a breech position. This means that its feet or buttocks would enter the birth canal first, instead of its head, which makes labor longer and more difficult for the baby. A C-section is also performed when the mother's pelvis is extremely small; when there are infrequent or weak uterine contractions; when the baby is unusually large or small; when the placenta blocks the baby from being born (placenta previa); when the placenta separates too soon from the uterine wall and hemorrhage occurs; or when the umbilical cord is pushed out ahead of the infant, compressing the cord and cutting off blood flow. In addition, a cesarean is performed if the mother has toxemia, vaginal herpes (which could infect a baby born vaginally and lead to its death), or pelvic tumors that obstruct the birth canal. Your hospital stay after a cesarean section will be five days or more.

If you do not want to have natural childbirth—deliver your baby with no anesthetic or pain relievers—you may request medicines to help relieve the pain. Analgesics are used to help relieve the pain of contractions. Relaxants, such as Valium, may also be used. Anesthetics are substances that completely deaden feeling in part or all of your body. A general anesthetic, which puts you to sleep, is rarely used today in vaginal deliveries because it can cause breathing problems for the baby.

Regional anesthesics are used most commonly today. These anesthetics deaden pain in limited areas of your body but allow you to remain awake to help your baby be born. Spinal anesthesia involves a single injection directly into the spinal fluid in the lower back, to block the pain-carrying nerves. A "saddle block" is a spinal injection that deadens a smaller area. Epidural anesthesia consists of injections of small amounts of anesthetics near the spinal nerves several times during labor. Caudal anesthesia consists of one or more injections near the tailbone. Pudendal and paracervical blocks are injections through the walls of the vagina and near the cervix.

There is no right or wrong method of childbirth. The final decision should be between you and your doctor. However, anesthesia does have possible side effects. Painkillers or sleep-inducing drugs may cause weaker contractions, which means a longer labor. Anesthesia may also slow the baby's heartbeat and breathing.

After delivery, it takes about six weeks for your uterus to return to its normal size. You may feel afterpains for a few days while your uterus keeps contracting. These contractions feel like mild menstrual cramps. If you are breast-feeding, you may experience more cramping while you are nursing. You can begin light exercises at home, but exercises to tighten the abdominal muscles should wait until after your postpartum visit to your doctor.

If you have had an episiotomy, you may use a heat lamp or analgesic spray to relieve discomfort. Later, either in the hospital or at home, you may take sitz baths. This means that you simply sit in warm water for about twenty minutes. You can eat as soon as you feel up to it, but remember to continue the good nutrition habits you began while pregnant. Ask your doctor whether you should take showers or baths until the episiotomy heals.

If you have a boy, you will be asked whether or not you want him circumcised. Circumcision is a simple operation to remove the foreskin from the penis. The operation was once a routine medical procedure for male babies, thought to be necessary for cleanliness. Today, however, there is believed to be no medical need for routine circumcision.

Low birth weight or premature babies are placed in a special care nursery, where you and the father and grandparents may visit. Be prepared to see a very tiny baby, wrinkly and red, perhaps with feeding tubes and machines to check the heart and breathing. You should feel free to touch, stroke, and talk to your baby, which will help him or her feel closer to you, even though your baby is in an incubator.

Before you go home from the hospital, you will be asked for information for your baby's birth certificate. If you have chosen the baby's name, it can be included. The information is sent to the registrar of births, and you can get a copy of the birth certificate from the Bureau of Vital Statistics, either in your city or in the state capital. You will need a copy of the birth certificate when your child enters school. If you are placing your baby for adoption, an amended birth certificate will later be issued in the adoptive parents' names, and will be the certificate required for school and all other identification purposes.

If you are breast-feeding, you will feel more comfortable if you wear a nursing bra for support. During the first few days after birth, a liquid called colostrum will come out of your nipples. Colostrum contains substances that protect your baby from infection. True breast milk comes out about three days after your baby is born. It is blue-white and does not look like cow's milk. You may experience some discomfort when colostrum changes to milk, but you can relieve the discomfort by nursing your baby frequently or by expressing (squeezing your milk out by hand). *Do not use oral contraceptives (birth control pills) while you are breast-feeding.*

One disadvantage of breast-feeding is that you must be with your baby at mealtimes in order to feed him or her, and babies' mealtimes occur very frequently, day and night. If you are working or going to school, breast-feeding may not be possible for you. Do not feel guilty about this. Plenty of healthy babies thrive on infant formula. The choice should be what works best for you. Whatever feeding method you use, however, you should hold your baby while you are feeding it. Do not prop your baby in an infant seat or crib with a bottle. By holding your baby during feedings, you are satisfying your child's natural craving to be cuddled, and you are helping form the bond between parent and child that leads to trust and love.

Some points in favor of breast-feeding are that your milk is easy for your baby to digest; it contains substances that help protect your baby from infections; it reduces the possibility that your baby will have allergic reactions; it is always clean and at the right temperature; and it is ready to serve when your baby is hungry. In addition, breast-feeding is free; it uses the extra fat your body stored for this purpose during pregnancy and so helps you lose weight faster; and it may help your uterus return to its normal size more quickly. About half the babies born in the United States

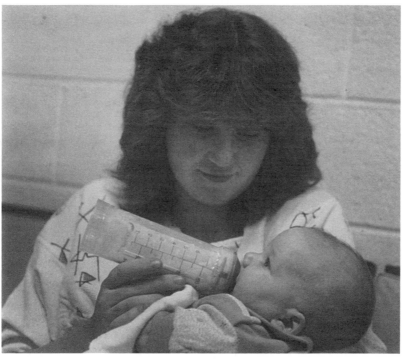

Babies quickly learn to recognize the touch, voice, and smell of the person who cares for them.

are now breast-fed. Breast-fed babies usually eat every two to three hours.

To produce an adequate supply of milk, you must eat even more essential nutrients than you did during pregnancy. Two extra servings of whole grains, or one additional serving of meat, fish, chicken, or dried beans plus an extra serving of raw or slightly cooked dark green leafy vegetables, or a serving of broccoli, tomatoes, cantaloupe, or watermelon will supply the extra nutrition you need. You will also need to drink eight to twelve glasses of liquids a day.

If you are not breast-feeding, wear a support bra and put ice packs on your breasts to reduce any discomfort you may feel. The swelling will usually disappear within thirty-six hours. Commercially prepared infant formulas, made from cow's milk or soy protein, are satisfactory alternatives to breast milk. However, they do not include the protective properties of breast milk. Formula-fed babies generally eat every three to four hours. You need to make sure the formula is comfortably warm by testing a few drops on your wrist. As the baby sucks, tilt the bottle so that its neck is always filled to prevent the baby from swallowing air. Remove the bottle occasionally to burp your baby and let him or her rest a minute or two.

During the first weeks after your baby is born, your body will be working to return to its pre-pregnancy condition. You may be constipated during this time, so eat plenty of high-fiber foods and raw fruits and vegetables, and drink plenty of water. Do not take strong laxatives if you are breast-feeding because they can give your baby diarrhea.

For about three weeks after delivery, you will have bleeding similar to a menstrual period. If the bleeding starts to smell bad or becomes bright red or heavy, let your doctor know. If you are breast-feeding, you may not menstruate for as long as you continue nursing. If you do not breast-feed, you will probably have your first period six to eight weeks after childbirth.

Usually you may resume sexual intercourse after four to six weeks; some doctors recommend that you wait until after your postpartum checkup, which is approximately six weeks after your baby is born. At that time, your uterus should be back to its normal size and position, and your weight may have dropped to about what it was before you became pregnant. The doctor will check your weight and blood pressure, test your blood for anemia, examine your breasts, perform a pelvic examination, and help you decide on a method of birth control.

Your ovaries begin producing eggs soon after delivery, even if you do not menstruate. *You can become pregnant.* Breast-feeding is *not* a foolproof contraceptive. For your own health and that of future babies, it is best to space your children at least eighteen months apart. Although you should not take oral contraceptives if you are breast-feeding, you may use other birth control methods. You can discuss these with your doctor.

Twenty-four hours after a normal delivery, with the approval of your doctor, you can begin to do exercises to strengthen your muscles and help you get back into shape. Lying on your stomach will help your uterus return to its normal position.

You will need a lot of rest and sleep when you come home from the hospital. Avoid heavy work for the first three weeks. The doctor will give you a list of things you can and cannot do for the first month or so after your baby is born. You may feel depressed a few days after giving birth. This is due to hormonal changes in your body, and will usually go away in a few days. Some women, however, even with adequate rest and nutrition, continue to feel depressed. This is called postpartum depression. You can ask your doctor to refer you to someone for help.

If you keep your baby, remember that you will also

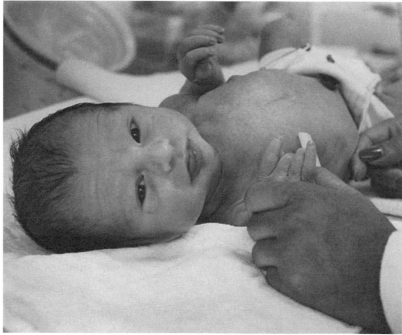

This newborn baby's wrinkles will soon disappear. Notice the stump of the umbilical cord above the diaper.

be adjusting to becoming a parent—not an easy job. Fitting a tiny baby into your daily routine takes time. Do not worry if some things do not get done as efficiently as they used to, or if you have to try out different ways of feeding, changing, burping, or bathing your baby. The only right way is what works best for you and your baby.

Remember, too, that newborn babies cry to make their needs known. Some cry more than others. You will soon be able to tell a hunger cry from a wet cry or a need-to-be-held cry. Sometimes a bath will soothe a crying baby. However, until the stump of the unbilical cord falls off (in about a week), give your baby only sponge baths. Use a sterile cotton ball to pat a little rubbing alcohol onto the area around and under the dried-out cord to keep the stump clean and help it to dry up. This will not sting the baby. If the baby cries, it is because the alcohol feels cold. If there is any bleeding or bad-smelling discharge from the cord or redness around it, report it to your doctor.

Shortly after you come home, phone your pediatrician (baby doctor) to schedule your baby's first checkup—usually when the baby is two to four weeks old. If you do not have a pediatrician, call your local health department, hospital, or county medical society and ask for a list of pediatricians, family practitioners, or clinics in your area. If you think your baby is not doing well at any time, phone your doctor or clinic.

No matter how old you are when you have a baby, seeing your baby being born is an unforgettable, incredible experience. As one girl says, "If you've never had a baby, nobody can tell you what it's like. You have to go through it yourself. I don't think there's anything else in the world that you can experience that will make you feel this happy. It's like if nothing good ever happened to you again in your life, seeing your baby being born would be enough."

SIX

Birth Control Methods and Saying No

THE MAJOR REASON for the many unplanned pregnancies each year is that couples do not use any form of birth control. For teenagers, often the reason is "I just didn't get around to it," or "I was afraid my parents would find out if I went to a birth control clinic." The truth is, however, family planning and Planned Parenthood centers offer confidential, free, or inexpensive birth control services. Your parents will not be notified, nor do you need their consent.

Recent studies show that five million American girls have had sex by the time they are seventeen, yet more than one-fourth of them have never used contraception. Eighty-eight percent of teenagers who seek birth control do so only after they are already sexually active. As a result, many become pregnant. Fifty percent of first pregnancies to unmarried teenagers occur within six months after they first have intercourse.

Many of these girls say they did not use birth control because they thought it was dangerous or because they were embarrassed or afraid to have a pelvic examination. Used properly, however, birth control methods are no riskier than being pregnant and having a baby. Moreover, some birth control methods help prevent sexually transmitted diseases. If you are not ready to have a baby, but are sexually active, some forms of birth control can offer you the security of relatively safe sex.

It is possible for a woman to become pregnant anytime she has sexual intercourse. Her partner's sperm cells can live in the woman's body and fertilize an egg for up to three days. Contraception (birth control) means preventing those sperm cells from uniting with an egg to form a baby—in other words, contraception means preventing pregnancy.

There are several methods of contraception. Some are available in drugstores without a prescription. Young people who use prescription methods, however, have a lower risk of becoming pregnant than those who use a nonprescription method.

One prescription birth control method is "the pill," or oral contraceptive. There are two types: combination pills and mini-pills. Both contain compounds similar to the hormones estrogen and progesterone produced by a woman's ovaries. Combination pills contain both hormones, and prevent a woman's ovaries from releasing eggs; mini-pills contain only progesterone, and create changes in a woman's cervix and uterus, making it difficult for sperm to meet and unite with an egg. Mini-pills are less effective. Each type requires a medical checkup, a pelvic examination, and a doctor's prescription.

Both types of birth control pills come in monthly packets. A whole packet must be taken day by day for the method

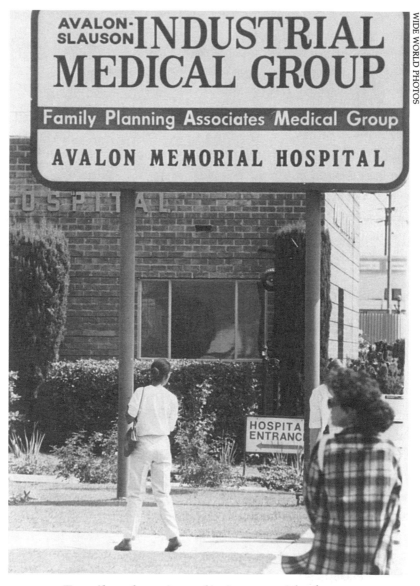

*Family planning clinics provide free or
inexpensive birth control services.*

to work. With twenty-one-day packs, you take pills for three weeks, then stop for a week, during which time your period usually occurs. The twenty-eight day packs and mini-pills are taken continuously. Protection continues as long as a pill is taken for the correct number of days each month.

If you forget a combination pill one day, take that pill and the next day's pill together. If you forget two combination pills in a row, take two pills on each of the next two days, but *also use an additional method,* such as a condom, a contraceptive sponge, or foam for the rest of that month in order to be fully protected. If you miss more than two pills, you may get pregnant. In that case, do not finish the packet, but instead use another method of birth control for the rest of your menstrual cycle. With mini-pills, skipping even one pill requires use of an additional method of birth control for the rest of the month.

Every form of birth control has its disadvantages. With the pill, chances of problems developing are greater for women over thirty-five, particularly if they smoke, are obese, or have diabetes or high blood pressure. For women under thirty, the health risks of the pill are much less than risks from pregnancy and childbirth. Some women experience morning sickness, which can often be reduced or eliminated by taking the pill with dinner or at bedtime. Other side effects may include tenderness or enlargement of the breasts, spotting between periods, weight gain or loss, and increased depression for women with a history of depression.

There are some serious side effects of taking the pill, though they happen very rarely. These include clots in the blood vessels of the legs, lungs, heart, or brain; heart attacks; and strokes. The chance of having these problems increases in women over thirty-five who have had blood vessel disorders. Heavy smoking (more than fifteen cigarettes a day) greatly increases the risk of serious side effects.

Serious problems related to the pill hardly ever develop without a warning. Signs to watch out for include yellowing of the skin or eyes; sudden or constant pain, redness, or swelling in the legs; pain in the abdomen, chest, or arm; shortness of breath; severe headaches; intense depression; or blurred vision. If these occur, call your doctor immediately.

There are several benefits from taking the pill, including some protection against benign breast tumors, ovarian cysts, and cancer of the ovaries. In addition, many women report that their periods are more regular, tension before their periods is lessened, and menstrual cramps are less painful. Some women on the pill have even said that acne and oily cysts on their faces have cleared up.

Of every one hundred women taking the pill, about two may become pregnant in the first year of use. If you decide you want to have a baby, you should stop taking the pill and use another form of birth control for about three months before trying to become pregnant. Of adolescents using some form of contraception, about 64 percent use the pill.

There is also a pill called the morning-after pill. However, this pill is an emergency measure only, and not for continued use. It is a high dosage of hormones, given as a series of pills that must be started within three days after one unprotected intercourse, during your midcycle. This pill may cause nausea and vomiting, and is only used in special circumstances, such as rape or incest.

A second type of birth control method that requires a

visit to a doctor is the diaphragm. This is a shallow cup made of rubber that is inserted into the vagina to cover the crevix, or opening of the uterus. Sperm-killing cream or jelly is smeared in the cup and around the rim before insertion. You insert the diaphragm before you have sexual intercourse. It works by blocking the entrance to the uterus, which prevents sperm cells from entering the uterus and combining with an egg cell. The sperm-killing cream immobilizes any sperm that might swim around the diaphragm rim.

Diaphragms come in different sizes, and your doctor will examine you to decide which size you need. He or she will show you how to insert the diaphragm at the same time. Your diaphragm size can change; it should be rechecked if you have a problem with the diaphragm slipping out of place, if you have had pelvic surgery or delivered a baby, if you have had a miscarriage or abortion, or if you have gained or lost a lot of weight.

You can insert the diaphragm two or three hours before intercourse. An additional application of cream or jelly must be used each time you have sex. The diaphragm should be left in place for at least six hours after the last act of intercourse. Do not douche until that time. Do not leave the diaphragm in for longer than twenty-four hours, as bacteria could form that might cause an infection and lead to toxic shock syndrome.

With proper care, a diaphragm should last about two years. Wash it with warm water and mild unperfumed soap. Let it air dry, then dust it lightly with cornstarch to keep the rubber flexible. Do not use Vaseline or scented bath powders, as these will weaken the rubber. Check the diaphragm every two or three months for holes.

A diaphragm offers some protection against sexually transmitted diseases and reduces the risk of developing cervical cancer and pelvic inflammatory disease. Rarely, women get a mild allergic reaction to the rubber of the diaphragm or to contraceptive jelly, which you can buy in a drugstore. Sometimes switching brands solves this problem. Some women may develop a bladder infection. Check with your doctor if you experience discomfort when the diaphragm is in place; irritation or itching in the genital area; or an unusual discharge from the vagina. Of one hundred women using the diaphragm, about nineteen become pregnant during the first year of use.

The cervical cap is similar to a diaphragm, but less than half the size. It also must be obtained from a doctor. It looks like a thimble and is made of rubber or plastic. Used with spermicide, the cervical cap fits over the cervix and blocks sperm from passing into the uterus. The cap can be worn for up to forty-eight hours, and while it is in place, it is unnecessary to use more spermicide before intercourse.

Women who use the cervical cap have a higher rate of abnormal Pap smears in the first few months of use. For this reason, the Federal Food and Drug Administration (FDA) recommends that the cap be prescribed only for women with normal Pap smears and that a Pap test be performed after three months of use. If that Pap smear is abnormal, use of the cap should be discontinued. Each year, out of one hundred women using the cervical cap, about fifteen become pregnant.

Another type of birth control that requires a medical examination—but one that is not usually recommended for adolescents—is the intrauterine device, or IUD. This is a small piece of plastic, usually with copper wrapped around the plastic, that is inserted into the uterus by a doctor and can remain there until a woman wants to become pregnant. The IUD keeps a fertilized egg from attaching to the lining of the uterus. It is usually inserted while you are having your period, as your cervix is softer at that time, which makes insertion easier. Only about five women in one hundred IUD users become pregnant during the first year. You should be aware, however, that because many women have had problems such as pelvic infections with the IUD, other methods of birth control are preferred today.

Several birth control products are available in drugstores without a prescription. The vaginal contraceptive sponge is one such product. The sponge is made of polyurethane foam that contains a sperm-immobilizing ingredient. It looks like a doughnut, with a depression, or "dimple," in the center, which fits over the cervix. It has a nylon loop across the bottom for easy removal. The sponge works by blocking the entrance to the uterus and by trapping and absorbing sperm cells, thereby preventing them from entering the uterus. The built-in chemical immobilizes sperm on contact.

Before sexual intercourse, you moisten the sponge with tap water, then insert it into the vagina. The sponge can be inserted up to eighteen hours before sexual intercourse, and can be left in the vagina and remain effective for up to twenty-four hours. The sponge should be left in place at least six hours after the last act of intercourse. It may be worn during swimming or bathing without losing its effectiveness, but it cannot be reused and should be thrown away after use.

Some women may be sensitive to the chemical in the

sponge. You should not use it if irritation, itching, or rashes occur. The sponge is not as effective as the pill, and there is also some concern that sponge users may be at risk for toxic shock syndrome (TSS). Because the sponge is a relatively new product, however, it is not known whether there is a definite relationship between TSS and sponge use.

To minimize the risk of TSS, do not use the sponge during menstruation, after delivery of a baby, or after an abortion, until the doctor says it is safe. Some warning signs to look out for are itching or irritation in the gential area; persistent unpleasant odor; or unusual discharge from the vagina. In addition, there is a rare risk of developing TSS if the sponge is left in longer than twenty-four hours. Of one hundred women using the sponge, nine to eleven will become pregnant.

Another non-prescription contraceptive is vaginal foam, a medicated mixture that looks and feels like aerosol shaving cream, and contains an ingredient that stops sperm activity. When inserted into the vagina before sexual intercourse, the foam spreads and covers the cervix, blocking the entrance to the uterus and killing sperm.

Foams come in aerosol containers with nozzles. The foam is inserted into the vagina with a narrow applicator that consists of a cylinder and a plunger, which should be inserted up to the top of the vagina. Then the plunger is pushed slowly to release the foam. Read the directions carefully before using. For most foam brands, you should shake the container at least twenty times. This causes bubbles to form. The more shaking, the more bubbles, and the more bubbles, the more the foam spreads out in the vagina to make a stronger barrier.

Foam is not as reliable as the pill. To be effective, it should be inserted just before intercourse, since the bubbles start going flat in about half an hour. A fresh application should be inserted before each sex act. Douching should be delayed for about six hours, to give the foam time to work fully. The applicator can be washed with warm water and mild soap. The chemical in the foam appears to provide some protection against certain sexually transmitted diseases and against pelvic inflammatory disease. Of every one hundred women who use foam, about eighteen become pregnant during the first year of use.

Combining foam with other contraceptive methods gives added protection against pregnancy—for example, using foam and a condom. You may use foam safely after childbirth, even if you are breast-feeding.

A word of caution: Often foam and feminine deodorants are displayed in drugstores side by side, and it is easy to mistake deodorant for foam. Make sure the word "Contraceptive" appears on the label.

A third non-prescription contraceptive is the condom, also called a rubber or prophylactic. The condom is shaped like the finger of a glove and is made of rubber or animal tissue. A man uses a condom by rolling it onto his erect penis before sexual intercourse. Its purpose is to catch sperm cells, preventing them from entering the vagina. A rubber condom should be discarded after one use. The condom is more effective if the woman at the same time uses vaginal contraceptive foam. Rubber condoms provide protection against sexually transmitted diseases, including AIDS. In one hundred couples using condoms, about ten pregnancies occur during the first year of use.

Birth Control Methods and Saying No

Some contraceptive methods are highly unreliable unless you follow them precisely. These are called fertility awareness methods (FAM). One is the withdrawal method, in which the man withdraws his penis from the vagina just before he reaches an orgasm, in order to keep sperm cells away from the uterine opening. The withdrawal method is unreliable because it requires a great deal of control from the man. Even then it is risky, since some sperm are released from the man's penis involuntarily before climax.

The other FAM method is periodic abstinence. This means that a couple avoids having sex during the time the woman is ovulating. Ovulation includes the days just before, during, and after an egg is released from the ovaries. To determine when this is likely to happen each month, the woman either takes her temperature every morning before getting out of bed or checks her mucus discharge daily. A doctor can instruct you on these procedures. These methods work only if you keep a very careful record. About twenty-four women out of every one hundred who use FAM become pregnant each year.

Some so-called birth control techniques *do not work at all.* They are douching, using plastic food wrap as a condom, and having sex during menstruation. For effective birth control, use one of the methods described in this chapter. Discuss the advantages and disadvantages of each method with your doctor before you decide which one to use.

Many teenage girls say they became pregnant because they believed certain myths about sex. Many others mistook sex for love.

For example, you may let yourself believe that if you

and your boyfriend want to have sex together, that must mean you two are in love. But it is normal to be "turned on" by someone without actually loving him. Two people can show they care about each other in a lot more ways than by having sex. Sharing your deepest feelings is one way, or being there to listen when the other person is hurting. If you are not sure that what you feel for a boy is love, ask yourself this question: "Are you hearing love when your body is saying sex?"

A variation of "sex equals love" is the notion that if a girl has sex with a boy, he will be more likely to love her. Yet people can have sex without love, and love can exist without sex. Often the first attraction a person feels to the opposite sex is physical. The love part takes time, and comes with getting to know the other person and discovering interests and values in common. In other words, when you think a boy is a "hunk," find out if his values and his mind live up to his body. When you are turned on by the way someone thinks, feels, cares, and communicates with you, there is a better chance for love to develop between the two of you than if the turn-on is mostly how the other person looks.

Often teenage girls do not use birth control because they believe if they use some form of contraception, they are in effect having planned sex. And to them, planned sex is not morally acceptable. If they are swept off their feet sexually, however, that is spontaneous, unplanned sex, which is okay. Translated into words, this is the "I couldn't help myself" type of sex.

Some girls believe (often because a boy has told them so) that if a boy is sexually aroused and doesn't climax, he will suffer painful physical problems, and therefore the girl must have sex with him at that point in their lovemaking in order to spare him pain. This is simply not true.

In fairness, it must be said that teenage boys also have some misconceptions about sex. For example, some boys believe that males have a stronger sex drive than females. This is not true. People of both sexes can have strong sex drives. Other boys believe that they have to have sex with several different girls in order to become better at making love. A girl usually responds to a boy who cares about her feelings, regardless of how sexually experienced he is.

Some boys mistakenly believe that if they have not had sex before they are sixteen, there must be something wrong with them. There is no official sexual rite of passage, and therefore, no age limit for a first sexual experience. And many boys believe that girls want to have sex but are unwilling to admit it. Therefore, these boys think that when a girl says no, she really means yes, and just wants to be talked into having sex. The truth is no one, boy or girl, wants to be pressured into having sex.

And both boys and girls often have sex because they believe "everyone is doing it." The fact is that almost half the teenagers in the United States are *not* "doing it." Moreover, in order to be "in," some teenagers will claim to have had sex when they have not. The argument that "everyone is doing it" is often used by one person to get another person to have sex. When one girl was told this line by a boy, she answered by saying, "Since everyone is doing it, you should have no trouble finding someone else to do it with."

Helen, fifteen, was extremely angry at her boyfriend when she unexpectedly became pregnant, because, as she says, "I wanted him to use a condom, but he said it wouldn't be as good for him if he did. I was so mad when I got pregnant. Look what I'm going through so he could have a few minutes of pleasure. I wish guys could get pregnant and see what we go through."

Angela, fourteen, reports, "I asked my boyfriend about using a condom, or my getting the pill, but he said, 'Oh, it'll be okay.' No, it won't be okay. Not when you get pregnant. Guys try to talk you into sex. Girls think about contraception more. Guys don't have to worry about it."

And Laurie, seventeen, says, "If I could do it over again, I'd plan ahead and be prepared with some kind of birth control. Or else I'd tell the boy to use a condom or forget it. Don't rush into sex with your eyes closed. Use contraception. Most boys will duck out and break up with you if you get pregnant. My boyfriend did. Boys should have to share some of the responsibility if their girlfriend gets pregnant. The baby is part of them, too, you know. But I guess guys can be irresponsible, because they don't have to have the baby. No way a girl can do that."

Everyone becomes ready for sex at different times. There is no set age at which a person should have sex. It is your decision, and you do not have to feel guilty or pressured into having sex before you are ready. If you are ready to have sex, but are not ready to have a baby, then using a reliable birth control method is one way to avoid becoming a parent too soon. When measured against the costs of an unwanted pregnancy, birth control by any method is worth working at. And the only method of birth control that is 100 percent reliable, has no side effects, and costs nothing is abstinence.

SEVEN

Sexually Transmitted Diseases

E ACH YEAR one American in twenty will contract a sexually transmitted disease (STD),
also called venereal disease (VD). Sexually transmitted diseases are passed from person to person through sexual contact. Of these diseases, there will be 2 million new cases of
gonorrhea; 80,000 of syphillis; 3 million of chlamydia; and
500,000 of genital herpes, which already afflicts more than
5 million Americans. Of the 1,004,029 cases of gonorrhea
reported in 1980, exactly 247,239 cases were in teenagers
age fifteen to nineteen, and it is estimated that 1 million
teenagers suffer from chlamydia each year. In fact, sexually
active teenagers are two to three times more likely to contract
STDs than people over twenty years old.

Fear, shame, and embarrassment have surrounded
STDs for centuries. There is often a feeling that only "dirty"
or "immoral" or "loose" people get STDs. The truth is, however, that anyone of any race, religion, social, marital, or
economic status can get STDs.

Many of the symptoms of sexually transmitted diseases
are similar, but treatment for each is different. Therefore, it

is important to see a doctor if you think you have an STD, so that proper treatment can be prescribed. Confidential testing and treatment are available in most communities. Ask your local Planned Parenthood center where to get help.

You *cannot* get a sexually transmitted disease from sitting on toilet seats or touching doorknobs in public rest rooms. If you have had an STD in the past and been cured, you *can* get it again. There are no vaccines against STDs, and the risk of infection will increase enormously if you have sex with a number of different people. Some forms of STD show few or no symptoms, so the infected person does not know that he or she has the disease and is spreading it. And it is possible to have more than one such disease at the same time.

STDs can infect men, women, and children. A pregnant woman can infect her unborn child. In women, these diseases cause, among other ailments, pelvic inflammatory disease (PID). In PID the fallopian tubes, uterus, cervix, and ovaries can become diseased, causing an increased risk of ectopic (tubal) pregnancy. PID causes pain, which interferes with an active, healthy life, and it can cause sterility in both men and women.

Gonorrhea and syphilis used to be the most common venereal diseases. Today, however, there are over twenty organisms recognized as being sexually transmitted. Here are some of the major STDs.

CHLAMYDIA

Chlamydia is one of the most rapidly increasing forms of VD in the United States. Chlamydia are organisms that cause a variety of infections if left untreated. In women, chlamydia causes PID. In both men and women, chlamydia can cause arthritis and infections in the urethra (the opening through which urine passes) and the eyes. A woman with PID sometimes needs later surgery to have damaged organs removed.

Symptoms of chlamydia include slight discharge; painful intercourse for women; burning urination; and urinating more often than usual. However, there may be no symptoms in 75 percent of all cases. If a pregnant woman has chlamydia, her baby's eyes may be infected during passage through the birth canal, or the baby may contract pneumonia, which may be fatal. Treatment is taking tetracycline, an antibiotic, or the antibiotic erythromycin if you are pregnant.

GONORRHEA

In women, gonorrhea may lead to PID or sterility; in males, it may cause problems in getting an erection and blocking of the urethra; and in both men and women, gonorrhea may cause heart disease, arthritis, eye diseases, blindness, and nervous system disorders. Pregnant women can infect their babies during birth. When a mother's water breaks before delivery, the bacteria can reach her baby's eyes, causing serious infection and possible blindness. To prevent this, all babies born in hospitals are treated promptly with medicated eye drops.

There are no symptoms of gonorrhea in 80 percent of women and in some men. In females, the infection is in the cervix. It may cause a green or yellow-green discharge; a mushroomlike odor from the genital area; pains in the abdomen, pelvic area, or shoulders; swelling and tenderness near the opening of the vagina; a burning sensation when urinating; a need to urinate more often than usual; and pus or blood in the urine. In males, gonorrhea occurs in the urethra, where it causes a puslike discharge and pain during urination.

Treatment for gonorrhea is a series of penicillin shots. However, a strain of gonorrhea that is resistant to penicillin has recently developed. Another antibiotic is used to treat this strain of the disease.

SYPHILIS

Syphilis is one of the most serious STDs, since it is life-threatening to men and women, and to any future children a woman may have. It is caused by an organism called a spirochete. The organism dies outside the human body and is killed by soap and water if present on the skin, which is a good reason for washing genital areas after sex.

There are four stages of syphilis when the disease is left untreated. In the first stage, a sore called a chancre—a painless, open, moist blister—appears on the genitals. In women, it usually appears on the cervix or the vagina, hidden from view. In men, it appears on the penis. Chancres may also appear, however, on the lips, in the mouth, or around the rectum. The highly infectious spirochete organism oozes from the chancre, which heals, with or without treatment, in one to five weeks.

The second stage of syphilis occurs from six to twenty-five weeks after the first stage. Symptoms usually include a general feeling of ill health; headaches; muscle or joint pains; loss of appetite; nausea; constipation; and a fever that hangs on over a period of time. Hair may fall out in patches. A very contagious rash may appear anywhere on the body, but is most often found on the outer skin of a woman's vagina. The rash develops into sores that ooze a clear fluid containing the infectious spirochete. Wartlike lesions may also appear on the genitals. Without treatment, the second stage usually passes in four to twelve weeks.

The third stage of syphilis is called the latent stage, meaning "quiet" or "hidden," and is divided into early and late latent syphilis. The third stage has no symptoms and is not infectious during sexual contact. However, a pregnant woman can pass the disease to her unborn baby, causing stillbirth or birth defects. Early latent syphilis lasts less than four years, and late latent syphilis from four years until the development of late syphilis.

The fourth stage of this disease, if it occurs, is called late syphilis. Symptoms for late syphilis are tumors in any affected organ; crippling paralysis; blindness; heart disease; brain damage; and death. Treatment consists of long-acting penicillin, or other antibiotics if the person is allergic to penicillin.

HERPES SIMPLEX VIRUS

Herpes simplex is caused by a virus. There are two forms: herpes simplex virus Type I, which affects the head and neck, causing cold sores or fever blisters; and herpes simplex Type II, which affects the genital area. Type I can also affect the genital area, usually as a result of having oral or anal sex with someone who has Type I.

People can spread herpes by touching an active sore in one part of the body and then touching another place on the body. You can take some precautions against spreading herpes: never touch the sores; always wash your hands after going to the bathroom; wash your hands before rubbing your eyes; and never moisten your contact lenses by putting them in your mouth.

The herpes virus remains in the body. Stress or illness can cause symptoms to recur. The first outbreak usually heals in ten to twelve days. Later outbreaks heal faster and are usually less painful. Sexual contact is not necessary for the disease to break out again.

Women infected for the first time with Type II may have no symptoms. Or they may have painful, fluid-filled blisters on the body, vagina, or cervix. The blisters break open and form painful, open sores. In men, the blisters usually occur on the penis or the urethra. A possible link has been found between gential herpes infection and, years later, cancer of the cervix.

A herpes infection during pregnancy increases the risk of miscarriage, stillbirth, or serious mental or physical damage to the baby as it passes through the birth canal. That is why a cesarean section is often done on women with active herpes infections. There is no cure for herpes. However, a new prescription drug called Zovirax has become available in ointment and tablet form. It can lessen the severity of the symptoms and shorten the length of the first outbreak.

Sexually Transmitted Diseases

AIDS

The newest sexually transmitted disease is Acquired Immune Deficiency Syndrome (AIDS), a fatal illness. AIDS is an abnormal condition in which the body's immune system (its ability to fight disease) is weakened. As a result, people with AIDS often develop serious infections and diseases that would not be a threat to anyone whose immune system was functioning normally, but which are often fatal to the AIDS patient. These are called "opportunistic" infections or diseases.

For example, about 82 percent of AIDS patients have had one or both of two rare diseases: a parasitic infection of the lungs called pneumocystis carinii pneumonia and a type of cancer known as Kaposi's sarcoma (KS). KS usually occurs on the surface of the skin or in the mouth. In early stages, it may look like a bruise, or a blue-violet or brownish spot. The spot persists and may grow larger. KS may spread to other organs of the body.

Other opportunistic diseases occurring in people with AIDS are toxoplasmosis, caused by a parasite that can infect the brain and the central nervous system and cause pneumonia; extreme diarrhea caused by an intestinal parasite; a fungus that coats the intestinal tract and is seen most often in the throat as hard, white patches of growth; cytomegalovirus (CMV), a viral infection of the digestive tract; herpes simplex; spinal meningitis; and lymphoma, a cancer which, in AIDS patients, affects the brain.

AIDS was first recognized in 1981. By 1987, the Public Health Service had received reports of more than 47,000 cases, about 52 percent of which had already resulted in death. An estimated 1.5 million other people have been infected by the virus that causes AIDS, but these people have no symptoms of illness. Scientists have discovered the virus that causes AIDS—human T-lymphotropic virus, type III (HTLV-III), also called human immunodeficiency virus (HIV). Because this virus continually develops new structures, it is difficult for scientists to study it and to develop a medical treatment.

Symptoms include tiredness, light-headedness, dizziness, headaches, unexplained rapid weight loss (10 pounds or more), persistent fevers, night sweats, dry cough, shortness of breath, and diarrhea. These symptoms may be accompanied by a thick white coating on the tongue or in the throat (thrush); swelling or hardening of glands located in the throat, groin, or armpit; the appearance of hard purplish growths on the skin or inside the mouth; a tendency to bruise more easily than usual; and unexplained bleeding from any body opening.

Tests are used to determine if a person's immune system is normal. In one, a small amount of blood is drawn and examined under a microscope to see if a certain type of white blood cell, which protects the body against disease, is present. The other test is performed by injecting a substance called an antigen under the skin. If a swelling or bump appears at the point of the skin test injection, this indicates that the person's immune system is healthy.

There is also a test for antibodies (substances produced in the blood to fight disease organisms) to HTLV-III. Presence of HTLV-III antibodies means that a person has been infected with that virus; it does not tell whether the person is still infected. The antibody test is used to screen donated blood and plasma and to assist in preventing cases of AIDS resulting from blood transfusions or use of blood products such as Factor VIII, needed by patients with hemophilia.

AIDS is spread by a blood-borne virus and is transmitted by sexual contact, intravenously through shared needles for drug injections, or by blood transfusions. People at greatest risk for AIDS include, in order of frequency: persons who are, or who have recently been, sexually intimate with homosexual or bisexual male partners; persons who have recently shared needles for the injection of drugs; persons who receive blood transfusions from donors who have AIDS; persons who have intimate contact with persons with AIDS, with the sexual partners of persons with AIDS, or with the sexual partners of persons who are at risk for AIDS; infants born to infected mothers. Pregnant women with AIDS virus are likely to give the disease to their unborn babies. AIDS is fatal to children born with the disease. Breast-feeding may also spread AIDS from mother to child.

The time between infection with the HTLV-III virus and the onset of symptoms ranges from six months to five years, and possibly longer. Not everyone exposed to the AIDS virus develops AIDS. These people may carry the virus for many years following exposure to it, but never develop any symptoms. People exposed to the AIDS virus who do not develop a full-blown case of AIDS may develop a less life-threatening condition called AIDS-Related Complex (ARC).

There is no evidence to suggest that a person can get AIDS from donating blood, or from daily nonsexual contact with those who have AIDS. Thus, you cannot get AIDS by shaking hands with someone who has the disease or by touching things people with AIDS have touched, such as doorknobs, bed linens, clothing, towels, toilets, telephones, showers, swimming pools, eating utensils, or drinking glasses. Neither can you get AIDS if a person with AIDS breathes, coughs, or sneezes near you.

Although the AIDS virus has been found in saliva and tears, there have been no cases in which exposure to either was shown to result in transmission of the disease. Thus, it is impossible to get AIDS by crying with, sweating with, kissing, or hugging people with AIDS. In practically all cases, direct sexual contact and the sharing of drug needles has led to the disease.

Currently, there is no cure for AIDS. Treatment at this time is focused on treating secondary illnesses that take advantage of the weakened immune system. Pneumocystis carinii pneumonia, for example, can be treated with antibiotics.

The National Institutes for Health and the Centers for Disease Control report that millions of Americans have already been exposed to the AIDS virus. About one in every thirty men between the ages of twenty and fifty may already carry the virus. These health centers project that in the next several years, the number of people in this country with AIDS will rise to hundreds of thousands.

Worldwide, as many as 10 million people are believed to be AIDS carriers, and according to some estimates, 100 million could have the virus by the end of this century. The U.S. government has targeted AIDS as its number one public health priority, and has established funding for research programs designed to develop vaccines and cures. If you want more information about the AIDS virus, there is a toll-free AIDS hot line: 1-800-342-AIDS.

To avoid getting AIDS or other STDs, take steps to ensure safer sex before you have sex. In particular, insist that your boyfriend use rubber condoms. Next, have sexual intercourse with only one person, and make sure that person is having sex only with you. Do not have sex with anyone who has been exposed to a sexually transmitted disease; have a physical examination to make sure you are free of STDs. Do not douche after sex, as douching may cause germs to go deeper into the cervical canal; and do not use your boyfriend's toothbrush, razor, or any other personal item that could be contaminated with blood.

EIGHT

Getting On with Your Life

WHETHER YOU HAVE chosen to have an abortion, to give up your child for adoption, or to raise your child, being pregnant has probably made a great impact on your life. In thinking about the future, many teenage girls say the most important goal for them is to finish their education.

"Whatever you do, stay in school," says fifteen-year-old Paula. "Without a high school diploma, you can't get a good job. And believe me, it costs a lot of money to raise a child, to live in a decent place, and to be able to buy extra things, not just the things you need to survive.

"I went to an alternative school for pregnant teenagers, because everyone there was going through the same problems I was. And the teachers really care about you and help you if you don't understand something. Also, at the alternative school you learn job skills like typing, accounting, and data processing, so you'll have that much more going for you when you apply for a job. And after your baby is born, the alternative school has a nursery where you can leave your baby while you are in class."

Like Paula, you may be able to find an alternative school in your community by asking your school counselor or a social worker at your state employment office. If there is no alternative school in your area, you can get a home tutor, go to night school, or attend adult education classes.

Today, more and more cities, however, have school programs in which pregnant teenagers can learn about prenatal care, childbirth, postnatal care, parenting, budgeting, and job skills for clerical, secretarial, and business positions. You can explore career choices and job skills while continuing your education in the basic subjects of science, math, English, and social studies.

Some of the job skills offered by alternative school programs are accounting and data processing, with which you can become a clerk, bookkeeper, or accountant; early childhood education, to prepare you to work in a day care center; and health occupations skills, to help you become a laboratory or X-ray technician, a nurses' aide, or a dentist's or doctor's assistant. Other vocational programs offer training in horticulture, landscaping, floral design, radio and television, agriculture, computer operation and programming, cosmetology, electronics technology, and technical drawing.

Another option is to get a high school General Equivalency Diploma (GED) by taking a test that covers your knowledge of English, math, history, and science.

Most teenage girls who have gone through an unplanned pregnancy also say the experience made them do some unplanned growing up. They usually have some definite thoughts about how being pregnant changed their lives, what they want to do in the future, and what they would do if they could go back in time to before they became pregnant. Here are some of their thoughts:

"I used to love to party every weekend with my friends," says Tina, age sixteen. "That all changed when I got pregnant. My boyfriend got real mad at me, like he thought getting pregnant was all my fault. He even said the baby wasn't his. Can you believe it? Then the kids at school acted like I was some kind of freak. It was like they didn't want to be seen with me, or they thought being pregnant was catching. And my friends stopped asking me to go out with them. I missed out on a lot. I never went to a prom. I missed all the parties and football games. I keep thinking, 'I'm just sixteen. I should have my whole life ahead of me to do anything I want.' But I can't do anything I want because I have a baby to take care of. I didn't realize how much I'd miss out on until I got pregnant."

Like Tina, fourteen-year-old Holly found being pregnant meant giving up some activities she enjoyed. "Before I got pregnant, I was on a gymnastic team. My dream was to make it to the Olympics. No way now. The really dumb thing is I wasn't even in love with the baby's father. I'd hardly dated at all, because I'd been so busy practicing gymnastics seven days a week. I'd only been out with this guy a couple of times. One night we went to a party, and everyone was drinking. They kept saying, 'Come on, Holly, have some.' I don't know why I listened to them. I guess I wanted them to like me. I got drunk, and I don't remember too much after that, except I got pregnant.

"My parents wanted me to get an abortion, but I just couldn't do it. So I quit the team, because there's no way you can walk on a balance beam or swing around parallel bars and be pregnant. Giving up gymnastics was hard. It was also hard to give up my baby for adoption. But I think it was the best thing for her.

"As for gymnastics, I'm all out of shape from being pregnant, and everyone on the team is so far ahead of me now, anyway. If I could go back to a year ago and change things, I'd never do anything where I didn't know what I was doing, like drinking too much, and ending up having sex with someone I didn't love, and getting pregnant."

For Beth, seventeen, both her social life and her home life changed drastically when she became pregnant. "My folks were so mad they wouldn't even talk to me. So I lived at a maternity home while I was pregnant. The bad part was there were all these rules at the home. I couldn't do what I wanted to when I wanted to anymore. The whole day we were on a schedule. We went to an alternative school until noon. Then after lunch we had prenatal and childbirth classes, and meetings with our social workers. Then we had about an hour free before dinner, and afterward we had to go to group therapy, which is this kind of rap session led by one of the social workers, where a bunch of us girls talked about being pregnant and whether we would keep our babies or not.

"When you live at a maternity home, if you want to go anywhere, you have to get a pass and be in by eleven. Most of the time, you have to go in a group and have one of the counselors along. That was really a drag. But the good part was being with other girls who were in my position, and talking about our plans for the future. Plus the people at the maternity home told me about places to apply for a

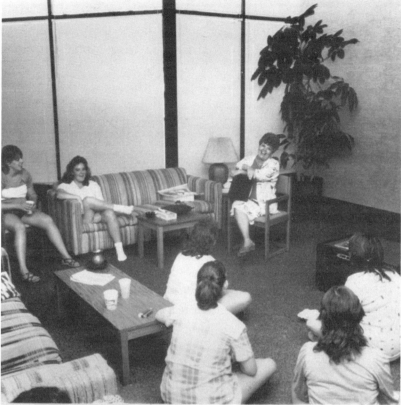

These pregnant teenagers enjoy one another's company at the Edna Gladney Maternity Home in Fort Worth, Texas.

job after my baby was born, and what schools had special classes for teenagers with babies, and about how to apply for money to buy food for me and my baby.

"Right now I'm sharing an apartment with three other girls and their babies. We take turns baby-sitting and chip in for food. I love my son, and I'm really glad I have him. But if I had it to do over again? No. I'd wait until I was older. Raising a baby is hard. You just can't imagine how hard it is until you try it."

Another girl has similar feelings. "When you think about having a baby, you think about how great it will be to have someone to love you who is all yours. What you don't think about is getting up at two A.M. to feed the baby, changing all those dirty diapers, and about how babies cry for hours sometimes, until you think you can't stand being a mother one more minute."

"I'm only fifteen," another girl says. "I want to do things other teenagers do. I'm a mother, but when I look at my own mom, I don't think I'm a parent yet. I was just learning how to be responsible for my own life. Then I got pregnant, and I had to stop thinking about myself and start being responsible for my baby and her life."

Fifteen-year-old Elaine has this advice: "Think about all your options—adoption, abortion, keeping your baby. Think it through and decide what would be the best for you and your baby. Remember, you're bringing a life into the world. It's not easy."

Lucy, seventeen, wanted to get pregnant because, she says, "I wasn't getting along with my folks. We argued all the time. I thought getting pregnant would help. But all I did was trade one bad situation for another. At least before the baby, I could go off by myself if I wanted to get away from problems for a while. But now I can't do anything without thinking of my baby first."

Another girl comments, "Some of my friends think having a baby will make people notice them, or their boyfriend be there for the rest of their lives, or their parents love them. That's not the way it works. You're really on your own when you have a baby. It doesn't make anyone love you. Other girls think having a baby will give them something of their very own to care about. They never turn around and see that they have themselves."

Terry, sixteen, has this to say about sex in general: "Having sex just because your friends are doing it, or because your boyfriend wants to, is no reason to have sex. You have to think about what can happen to you. Boys don't have to worry about getting pregnant when they're pushing you to have sex with them. Maybe you're just not ready to have sex, even if your friends are. It took getting pregnant for me to realize there's nothing wrong with saying no."

Janet, also sixteen, has similar feelings. "If I had it to do over again, I'd date a lot of different boys, instead of just one. I'd really get to know a guy before having sex with him. I'd want to know how he felt about certain things. Then I'd be able to know if he really cared about me, or if he was just out for sex."

Another girl adds, "It's been six years since I had my baby, and I've finally met a guy who really loves me. It makes all the difference in the world. When I look back, I can't believe I ever settled for anything less."

Terry and Janet are right. If you have already had sex with one person, or even if you've had a baby, there is nothing wrong with waiting to have sex again until you are ready. You have to decide what *you* want and what is best for *you*. Nobody else can, or should, make that decision for you, including your boyfriend. Everyone has different feelings, needs, and values. Therefore, it makes sense that how another person feels about sex may not be the way you feel about it.

Sometimes people have sex for reasons that have little to do with loving the other person. Perhaps they believe having sex with someone will make them feel less lonely or unhappy; or they believe having sex will make them more popular. Boys sometimes believe that having sex with many different girls will prove they are macho; and girls frequently use sex as a way to prove their independence from their parents, or to get back at their parents when they are angry with them. Teenagers of both sexes often believe that having sex will make them grown-ups.

Having sexual intercourse will not make you an adult, solve your problems, or change unpleasant situations. In fact, it may even make matters worse if you become pregnant or get a sexually transmitted disease. Raising a child is a 24-hour-a-day, 365-day-a-year job for about twenty years. If you are uncertain of your feelings about sex, it is okay to say no and keep saying no until you are sure. You do not even have to give the other person a reason, or you may give an explanation you feel comfortable with, such as, "I like you a lot, but I've decided to wait awhile," or "Sex isn't something I want to deal with yet."

The decisions you make about sex and motherhood will depend on what you want your life to be like. What kind of career do you want? How much further education do you hope to have? Are there other things you dream of doing? Will having a baby interfere with achieving your goals? The more sure you are of yourself and what you want to attain in life, the less likely you are to be pushed into doing something you do not want to do.

When thinking about whether having sex is right for you at a particular time, here are some questions you might ask yourself:

"If I get pregnant, can I handle getting an abortion, being a mother, or giving my baby up for adoption?"

"Can I support a child, financially and emotionally?"

"Am I sure no one is pushing me into having sex?"

"If I break up with this person, will I be glad I had sex with him?"

Dorothy had a baby when she was nineteen. She has this to say about the experience five years later: "Before my baby was born, I thought all you did for babies was put cute clothes on them, feed them, change them, and put them to bed. I used to think babies were so cute and wish I had one, because it would be so much fun taking care of a baby.

"Now I've got one, and let me tell you babies are not cute or fun a lot of the time. You have to do a lot more than feed, change, and dress them. When they get older, you have to teach them how to feed themselves, go to the bathroom by themselves, and dress themselves. You have to teach them right from wrong, to be nice to other people, and things like don't run in the street or touch a hot stove. They're always into something, and you better not leave them alone for a second if you don't want things torn up around your house or your child to get hurt.

"Lots of girls think being a mother comes naturally just because you're a girl. But you have to learn how to be a mother. You're not born knowing how."

Karen, eighteen, talks about life as a single teenage parent, saying, "The bad part is that your friends think you're too old for them, because you can't party anymore. They're out having fun, and you're stuck at home taking care of a baby. Of course, there's the good part. A baby is a part of you, and you love that baby no matter what. And there are good times when you're just so glad to have that baby to take care of, and it makes you feel so good taking care of it.

"But you also think maybe you should have waited a little longer before becoming a parent. I wasn't even thinking about having a baby when I got pregnant. My boyfriend talked me into having sex. I didn't stop to think it would be *my* life, not his, that would get messed up if I got pregnant. Now he's off in another town going to college, and I'm trying just to finish high school.

"If I could tell other girls one thing, it would be that when a guy says, 'If you loved me, you'd have sex with me,' you should say back, "If you loved me, you'd never say that.' I use birth control pills all the time now, whether I need to or not. I messed up once. I'm not messing up again."

Love and sexual feelings can be expressed in many different ways, only one of which is sexual intercourse. Hugging, kissing, touching, sharing, respecting each other's feelings, and treating each other with consideration and trust—all these and more are expressions of caring between two people.

When you think about whether to have a child, it is a good idea to think about what a child is. He or she is an individual person with feelings, not a hobby, or something whose duty is to make you feel loved. Babies cry when you're asleep and sleep when you're awake. They get sick and can't tell you what is wrong. They are totally dependent upon you for food, shelter, and care. Your problems do not go away when your children grow older; you will simply have different problems, such as worrying about their driving a car, or their college tuition.

The well-known author and humorist, Erma Bombeck, has written that "Parenting is like the domestic Peace Corps. The hours are long. The work is hard. The pay is zip. Giving birth is little more than a set of muscular contractions granting passage of a child from the uterus. Then, the mother is born."

Further Reading

Bode, Janet. *Kids Having Kids*. New York: Franklin Watts, 1980.

Hansen, Caryl. *Your Choice*. New York: Avon, 1980.

Hyde, Margaret O., and Elizabeth H. Forsyth, M.D. *AIDS: What Does It Mean to You?* Revised edition. New York: Walker, 1987.

Lerner, Ethan A., M.D., Ph.D. *Understanding AIDS*. Minneapolis, MN: Lerner Publications, 1987.

Lindsay, Jeanne Warren. *Pregnant Too Soon*. St. Paul, MN: EMC Publishing, 1980.

Lindsay, Jeanne Warren. *Teens Look at Marriage*. Buena Park, CA: Morning Glory Press, 1984.

Lindsay, Jeanne Warren. *Teens Parenting*. Buena Park, CA: Morning Glory Press, 1981.

McGuire, Paula. *It Won't Happen to Me*. New York: Delacorte, 1983.

Miner, Jane Claypool. *Young Parents*. New York: Julian Messner, 1985.

Nemiroff, Jane Libman. *Practicing Parenting*. New York: Butterick, 1980.

Nourse, Alan E., M.D. *AIDS*. New York: Franklin Watts, 1986.

Roggow, Linda, and Carolyn Owens. *Handbook for Pregnant Teenagers*. Grand Rapids, MI: Zondervan, 1985.

Sills, Barbara. *The Mother to Mother Baby Care Book*. New York: Avon, 1980.

Spock, Dr. Benjamin, *Baby and Child Care*. Revised edition. New York: Pocket Books, 1985.

Walsworth, Nancy, and Bradley Walsworth. *Coping with Teenage Motherhood*. New York: Rosen Group, 1979.

Appendix:
Organizations and
Agencies That Help
Pregnant Adolescents

Following is a list of organizations whose purpose is to help pregnant adolescents find programs in prenatal care, childbirth, and parenting; free or inexpensive birth control; help with staying in school, including day care facilities for infants and young children; low-cost medical care; sources for job opportunities; and assistance in locating housing, clothing, and infant supplies. *Note:* You do not have to live in the same state as a particular organization to phone or write them for assistance.

Alabama

Charles Henderson Child
  Health Center
P.O. Box 928
Troy, AL 36081
(205) 566-7600

Arizona

Associated Services for
  Adolescent Family Education
Tucson Unified School District
1010 East Tenth Street
Tucson, AZ 85717
(602) 628-7881

California

Saint Anne's Maternity Home
155 North Occidental Blvd.
Los Angeles, CA 90026
(213) 381-2931

Teen Advocate Program
South Bay Free Clinic
1807 Manhattan Beach Blvd.
Manhattan Beach, CA 90266
(213) 374-2149; 374-CARE (hot line)

Teen Mother Program
Tracy Educational Center
12222 Cuesta
Cerritos, CA 90701
(213) 926-5566, Ext. 2423

Teen Parent Assistance
Program
Oakland Unified School District
1025 Second Avenue
Oakland, CA 94606
(415) 834-8745

Information and Education
Program
San Diego Urban League
4261 Market Street
San Diego, CA 92101
(619) 263-3115

Teenage Pregnancy and
Parenting Project
1010 Gough Street
San Francisco, CA 94109
(415) 648-8810

Colorado

Urban League for the Pikes
Peak Region
324 North Nevada
Colorado Springs, CO 80903
(719) 634-1525

Child Opportunity Program
3607 Martin Luther King Blvd.
Denver, CO 80205
(303) 399-0603

Connecticut

Hill Health Corporation
400 Columbus Avenue
New Haven, CT 06519
(203) 436-7811

Rural Adolescent Pregnancy
Program
158 Main Street
Putnam, CT 06260
(203) 928-6567

Florida

School Board of Sarasota
County
2418 Hatton Street
Sarasota, FL 33577
(813) 953-5000

The Greater Tampa Urban
League, Inc.
1405 Tampa Park Plaza
Tampa, FL 33605
(813) 229-8117

Appendix

Junior League of Central and
North Brevard
442 Magnolia Avenue, #25
Merritt Island, FL 32952
(305) 453-5188

Economic Opportunity Family
Health Center, Inc.
5361 N.W. 22nd Avenue
Miami, FL 33142
(305) 835-8122

Georgia

Parent and Child Development
Services, Inc.
312 East 39th Street
Savannah, GA 31401
(912) 355-9475

Hawaii

Hawaii Adolescent Family Life
Project
761 A Sunset Avenue, Wilcox
Blvd.
Honolulu, HI 96816
(808) 735-3056

Illinois

New Horizons
Tri-County Urban League
317 South MacArthur Highway
Drive
Peoria, IL 61605
(309) 673-7474

Junior League of Chicago
1447 North Astor Street
Chicago, IL 60610-1698
(312) 664-4462

Hull House
118 North Clinton Street
Chicago, IL 60606
(312) 726-1526

Indiana

City of Gary Dept. of
Emergency Referral Services
Marion Home
1100 Massachusetts Street
Gary, IN 46407
(219) 886-3051

Iowa

Concerned United Birthparents
2000 Walker Street
Des Moines, IA 50317
(515) 263-9558

Kansas

Adolescent Family Life Services
Lyon County Health Dept.
802 Mechanic
Emporia, KS 66801
(316) 342-4864

Kentucky

Covington Family Health
Center
302 Court Street
Covington, KY 41011
(606) 491-7616

Maternal and Child Health
Center
12 East Fifth Street
Newport, KY 41071
(606) 431-1704

Louisiana

Office of Women's Services
200 Riverside Mall
P.O. Box 94095
Baton Rouge, LA 70804–9095
(504) 342-6029

Maine

Sisters of Charity Health
Systems
200 College Street
Lewiston, ME 04240
(207) 783-1021

Maryland

Saint Ann's Infant and
Maternity Home
4901 Eastern Avenue
Hyattsville, MD 20782
(301) 559-5500

Massachusetts

Teen Parent Family Support
Project
Dept. of Health and Hospitals
818 Harrison Avenue, HOB
#402
Boston, MA 02119
(617) 424-4556

Junior League of Holyoke
243 Maple Street
Holyoke, MA 01040
(413) 532-3640

Junior League of Springfield
254 Worthington Street
Springfield, MA 01103
(413) 734-3921

Michigan

Detroit Urban League
208 Mack Avenue
Detroit, MI 48201
(313) 832-4600

Teenage Parent Alternative
School Program
2000 Pagel
Lincoln Park, MI 48146
(313) 386-1250

Minnesota

Junior League of Minneapolis
1455 West Lake Street, Suite 318
Minneapolis, MN 55408
(612) 824-3271

Appendix

St. Paul–Ramsey Medical
  Center
640 Jackson Street
St. Paul, MN 55108
(612) 221-8876

Mississippi

Teen Parent Program
2906 North State Street
Jackson, MS 39216
(601) 366-0025

Missouri

Parent Infant Interaction
  Program
Vashon High School, Room 107
3405 Bell
St. Louis, MO 63106
(314) 531-9028

Urban League of St. Louis
Family Life Education Program
St. Louis Urban League
3701 Grandel Square
St. Louis, MO 63108
(314) 371-0040

Junior League of St. Louis
Teen Outreach Program
8346 Delcrest
St. Louis, MO 63124
(314) 872-1960

Junior League of St. Joseph
304 North Eighth Street
St. Joseph, MO 64501
(816) 232-4326

Montana

Young Families Program, Inc.
1001 North 30th Street
Billings, MT 59101
(406) 245-7328

Nebraska

Junior League of Omaha
7400 Court Building, Suite #102
Omaha, NE 68114
(402) 391-8986

New Hampshire

Home Health Agency of
  Greater Manchester
194 Concord Street
Manchester, NH 03104
(603) 622-3781

New Jersey

Family Life Program
Urban League of Metropolitan
  Trenton
209 Academy St.
Trenton, NJ 08608
(609) 393-1512

Camden County Dept. of
  Health
2101 Ferry Avenue
1800 Pavilion West
Camden, NJ 08104
(609) 757-4458

New Mexico

Adolescent Family Life
  Program
101 North Alaneda Blvd.
Las Cruces, NM 88005
(505) 523-2042

New York

Adolescent Health Center
Mount Sinai Hospital
19 East 101st Street
New York, NY 10028
(212) 650-7214 or 650-7215

Adolescent Health
Harlem Hospital
136th Street near Fifth Avenue
K Building, Room 343–345
New York, NY 10037
(212) 694-8223

Martin Luther King Clinic
50 Lenox Avenue at 112th Street
New York, NY 10026
(212) 876-6670

Maternity Infant Care
Family Planning
158 East 115th Street
New York, NY 10026
(212) 396-9500

William F. Ryan Community
  Health Center
Teen Health Project
160 West 100th Street
New York, NY 10025
(212) 678-5699

Maternity Infant Care
Family Planning
26 Old Broadway at 126th Street
New York, NY 10027
(212) 663-3992

Monroe County Adolescent
  Pregnancy Preventive and
  Supportive Services
Monroe County Health Dept.
111 Westfall Road, Caller 632
Rochester, NY 14692
(716) 442-4000, Ext. 2774

Junior League of Orange
  County
P.O. Box 515
Middletown, NY 10940
(914) 343-6095

North Carolina

Junior League of Greensboro
220 State Street
Greensboro, NC 27408
(919) 379-8226

Appendix

Adolescent Parent Prevention
  Program
Greene County Health Care,
  Inc.
P.O. Box 657
Snow Hill, NC 28580
(919) 747-5841

Ohio

Community Chest and Council
  of the Cincinnati Area
2400 Reading Road
Cincinnati, OH 45202
(513) 721-7900

Planned Parenthood of Central
  Ohio
206 East State Street
Columbus, OH 43215
(614) 224-2235, Ext. 212

Services for Unmarried Parents
  and Specialized Adoptions
  (SUMA)
1216 East McMillan
Cincinnati, OH 45026
(513) 221-7862

SUMA (Clermont County
  Office)
233 East Main Street
Batavia, OH 45103
(513) 732-6004

Single Parent 24-Hour Hot
  Lines
Hamilton and Clermont
  Counties: (513) 721-7900
Brown County: (513) 378-3027

Planned Parenthood
  Association of Butler County
11 Ludlow Street
Hamilton, OH 45011
(513) 856-8332

Jewish Family Service
1710 Section Road
Cincinnati, OH 45227
(513) 351-3680

March of Dimes
5041 Oaklawn Drive
Cincinnati, OH 45227
(513) 396-7500

Oklahoma

Salvation Army Maternity
  Home
Box 3303
Tulsa, OK 74101
(918) 245-1827

Oregon

Teen Mother Program
768 State Street
Salem, OR 97301
(503) 581-9922

Pennsylvania

Teen Pregnancy Intervention
  Program
Philadelphia Urban League
1930 Chestnut Street, Suite 200
Philadelphia, PA 19103
(215) 561-0700

Adolescent Pregnancy Program
Shenango Valley Urban League
314 Idaho Street
Farrell, PA 16121
(412) 981-5310

Junior League of Philadelphia
Free Quaker Meeting House
Fifth and Arch Streets
Philadelphia, PA 19106
(215) 923-6777

Maternal and Family Health
  Services, Inc.
37 North River Street
Wilkes-Barre, PA 18701
(717) 822-2325

Rhode Island

Project Birth
Urban League of Rhode Island
246 Prairie Avenue
Providence, RI 02905
(401) 351-5000

Ethnic Adolescent Family Life
  Project
469 Angell Street
Providence, RI 02906
(401) 861-6300

South Carolina

Saint Mary Human
  Development Center, Inc.
Route 1
Box 177
Ridgeland, SC 29936
(803) 726-3338

Tennessee

Appalachian Adolescent
  Health and Education Project
Douglas-Cherokee Economic
  Authority, Inc.
P.O. Box 1218
Morristown, TN 37816–1218
(615) 587-4500

St. Peter Home for Children
1805 Poplar Ave.
Memphis, TN 38104
(901) 725-8240

Texas

Comprehensive Adolescent
  Health and Education
  Program
Gulf Coast Council of La Raza
2203 Baldwin Street
Corpus Christi, TX 78405
(512) 881-9988

The Edna Gladney Home
2110 Hemphill
Fort Worth, TX 76110
(817) 926-3304

Appendix

Dallas Urban League
2121 Main St., Suite 410
P.O. Box 15492
Dallas, TX 75201
(214) 747-4734

Catholic Family Service, Inc.
1522 South Van Buren
P.O. Box 15127
Amarillo, TX 79105
(806) 376-4571

Utah

Teen Mother and Child
  Program
University of Utah Medical
  Center
50 North Medical Drive
Salt Lake City, UT 84132
(801) 581-3729

Vermont

Addison County Parent/Child
  Center
Box 646
Middlebury, VT 05753
(802) 388-3171

Virginia

Norfolk Adolescent Pregnancy
  Prevention and Services
Norfolk State University
School of Social Sciences
2401 Corprew Avenue
Norfolk, VA 23504
(804) 623-8651

Washington

Options for Pregnancy
P.O. Box 88007
Seattle, WA 98188
1-800-732-1887

Junior League of Yakima
5000 West Lincoln
Yakima, WA 98902
(509) 966-7174

Tacoma–Pierce County
  Adolescent Pregnancy
  Program
3629 D Street, FC: 3213
Tacoma, WA 98408
(206) 591-6401

Washington, D.C.

Single Teen Parent Training
  Program
Washington Urban League
3501 14th Street N.W.
Washington, DC 20010
(202) 265-8200

Adolescent Health Center
1325 W Street N.W.
Washington, DC 20009
(202) 861-0230

West Virginia

Youth Health Services
Memorial General Hospital
 Assoc., Inc.
1200 Harrison Avenue
Elkins, WV 26241
(304) 636-9450

Wisconsin

Teen Pregnancy Service
2711 Wells Street
Milwaukee, WI 53208
(414) 937-2727

Index

Index

About the Author

Herma Silverstein was born in Fort Worth, Texas. She graduated from Sophie Newcomb College of Tulane University in New Orleans, where she majored in Spanish. She has written both fiction and nonfiction books for young people, including *Anti-Semitism: A Modern Perspective* and *Hoaxes That Made Headlines*, both published by Julian Messner.

As part of researching *Teenage and Pregnant: What You Can Do*, Ms. Silverstein talked to over one hundred pregnant or parenting teenage girls throughout the United States. Although their names have been changed to protect their privacy, some of their experiences and advice is included in this book.

Ms. Silverstein lives in Santa Monica, California, with her two sons, Larry and Ben.